pure skin care

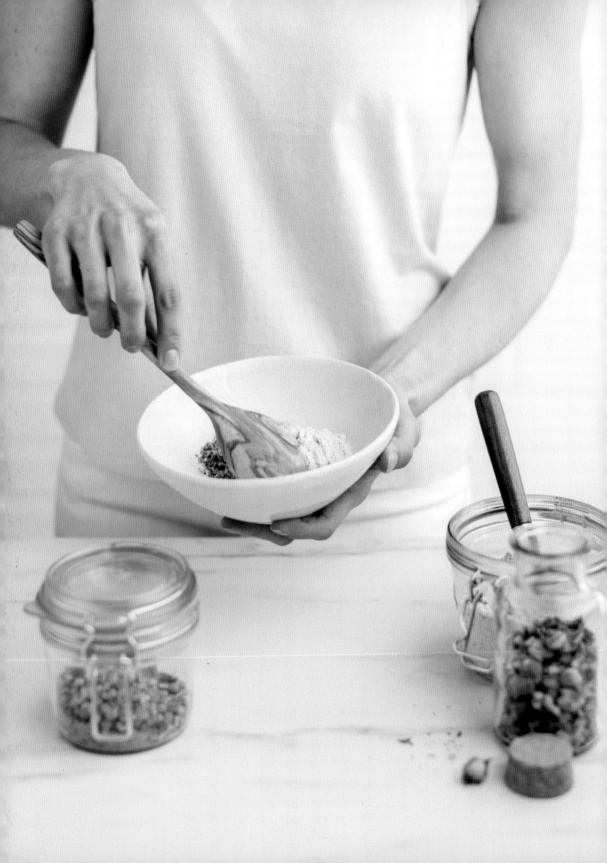

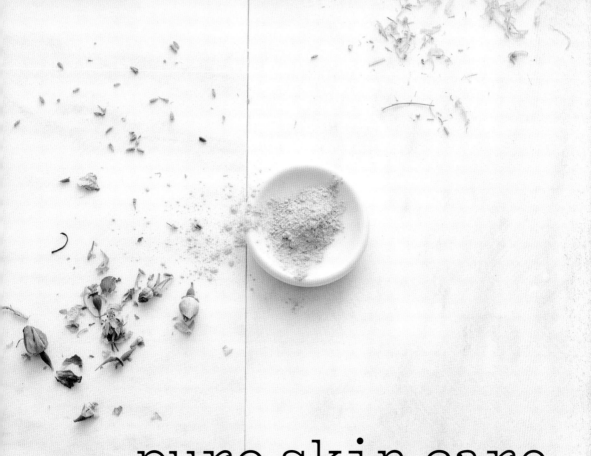

pure skin care

Nourishing Recipes for Vibrant Skin & Natural Beauty

Stephanie L. Tourles

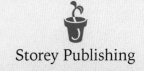

Storey Publishing

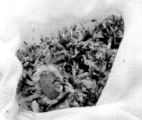

The mission of Storey Publishing is to serve our customers by publishing practical information that encourages personal independence in harmony with the environment.

Edited by Deborah Balmuth and Michal Lumsden
Art direction and book design by Michaela Jebb
Text production by Jennifer Jepson Smith
Indexed by Christine R. Lindemer, Boston Road
    Communications

Cover and interior photography by
    © Michael Piazza Photography
Photo styling by Darcy Hammer
Hair and makeup styling by Liz Washer/Ennis Inc.
Illustrations by © Babeth Lafon/@babethlafon/
    Illustration Division

This publication is intended to provide educational information for the reader on the covered subject. This book is not intended to replace professional medical advice or treatment. Read the instructions carefully and follow the safety precautions completely when making recipes.

Storey Publishing
210 MASS MoCA Way
North Adams, MA 01247
storey.com

Printed in China through Asia Pacific Offset
10 9 8 7 6 5 4 3 2 1

LIBRARY OF CONGRESS CATALOGING-IN-PUBLICATION DATA

Names: Tourles, Stephanie L., 1962– author.
Title: Pure skin care : nourishing recipes for vibrant skin
    & natural beauty / Stephanie L. Tourles.
Description: North Adams, MA : Storey Publishing, 2018.
    | Includes bibliographical references and index.
Identifiers: LCCN 2018012689 (print)
    | LCCN 2018014771 (ebook)
    | ISBN 9781635860511 (ebook)
    | ISBN 9781635860504 (hardcover with
    concealed wire-o : alk. paper)
Subjects: LCSH: Skin—Care and hygiene.
    | Herbal cosmetics. | Beauty, Personal.
Classification: LCC RL87 (ebook)
    | LCC RL87 .T69 2018 (print)
    | DDC 646.7/2—dc23
LC record available at https://lccn.loc
    .gov/2018012689

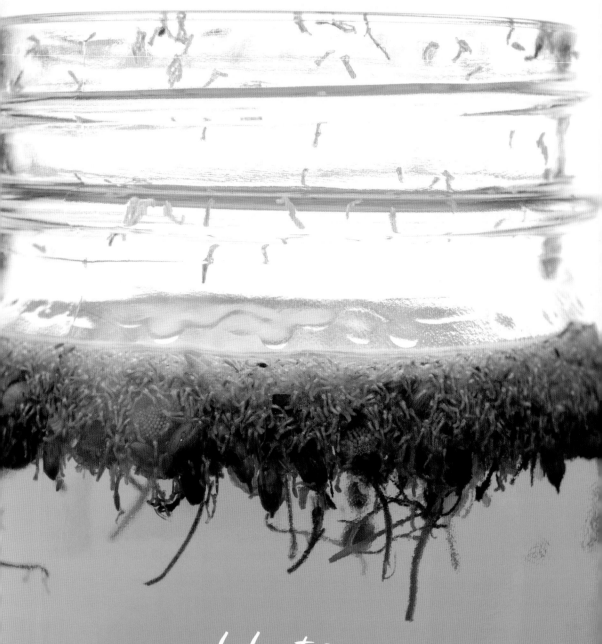

dedication

To my mother, Brenda Anchors

You taught me from a young age that following a good skin care regimen and using high-quality products would promote a complexion beaming with radiance. Now, in my late fifties, my skin positively glows with good health. Thanks, Mom!

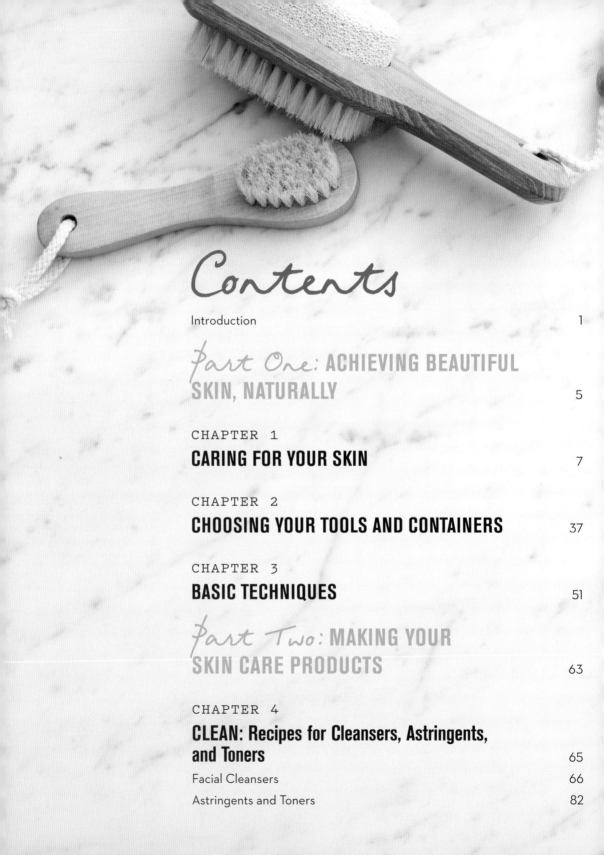

Contents

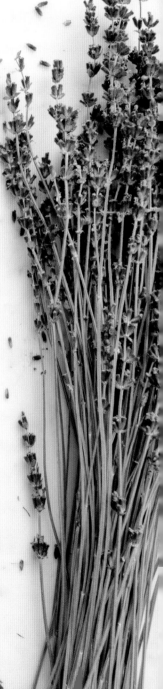

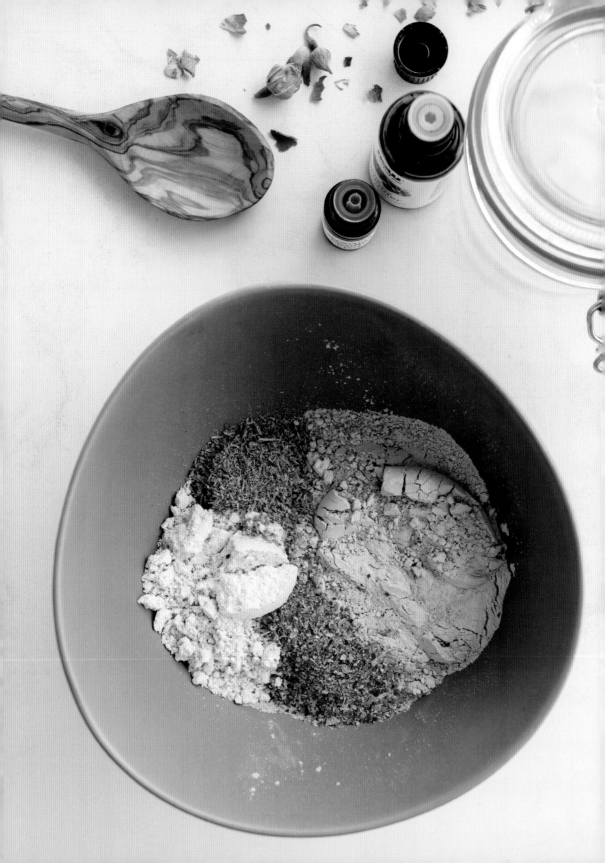

INTRODUCTION

Did you know that women use an average of 12 personal care products daily? And men aren't far behind, with about seven in their daily routine. Every day we use products such as soap, body scrub, lotion, face cleanser, toner, shaving cream, sunscreen, makeup, deodorant, and more. Our skin eats — or, more accurately, absorbs — up to 60 percent of whatever we put on it, so it's important to know what is in these products we are slathering on ourselves.

The official term for the process of absorption of substances via the skin is *transdermal penetration*. The degree to which a substance applied topically can penetrate the skin depends on the particular substance, the molecular size of its ingredients, the temperature, and the condition of the skin at the time of contact. If you're having a hard time believing that your skin can actually absorb some of the ingredients from your favorite body care product, then you have only to think of four popular drugs that are transported into the bloodstream via a topical patch: nicotine used for cessation of smoking, hormones for birth control, scopolamine for motion sickness, and nitroglycerin for angina pectoris.

As a licensed esthetician and holistic skin care specialist, my focus is on educating individuals so that they can realize their highest health and beauty potential through the use of natural skin and body care products and vitalizing lifestyle habits. I want my clients and readers to become active participants in their own well-being.

Over the years, I have worked with a wide range of commercial products, including high-end and "natural" products from health food stores and wellness spas. Many of these body care preparations, even the so-called natural ones, contain potentially toxic and irritating ingredients. I've heard from both clients and readers who endured allergic reactions or other skin sensitivities resulting from their use of these often costly and often synthetic-blend products.

On the flip side, if potentially irritating or harmful chemicals and artificial colorants and fragrances can be absorbed by your skin, then so can highly beneficial natural ingredients, which can promote beautiful, healthy skin.

In this rapidly advancing technological age of skin and body care, a dizzying array of "youthifiers" are available. While some of these technological advancements — such as acid-based skin peels, pharmaceutically enhanced cosmetics, microdermabrasion, and surgical face and body reconstruction — do have their place, they shouldn't prevent us from taking control of our own bodies. These quick fixes do not come without some pain, risk, or expense. Nor do they offer an everlasting cure-all to our perceived physical shortcomings.

The time is ripe for getting back to the basics. Many of us have lost sight of our true selves in an effort to become synthetically enhanced, smoothed, or physically augmented. It's important to remember, however, that Hollywood hype is not reality — nor should it be.

Holistic herbal skin and body care comprises an ancient tradition that promotes mutual respect between individuals and generations, harmony and balance within, gentle coexistence with the earth, and a visible physical radiance in the individuals who practice it. Herbs and other natural ingredients cleanse, protect, and pamper the skin; smell wonderful; and nourish both body and soul. They produce in us a profound sense of authentic beauty, contentment, and well-being.

With the instructions and recipes in this book, you'll learn how to create natural, often organic personal care products for skin, feet, and hands that sing with vitality, vibrance, and inner wellness. The formulas I've created will help correct current skin problems and prevent future ones as well as smooth and balance your skin.

As you'll learn, the consistent practice of holistic health, beauty, and lifestyle habits is always the key to looking and feeling your best. But don't forget to have some fun along the way, too. Whether you're new to making handmade personal care products or are highly skilled at cosmetic cookery, keep in mind that these recipes are designed to be relatively easy to make, pleasurable to use, and simple to customize according to your needs or whims. Many make great gifts, too.

May your journey with herbs and other pure, natural ingredients bring you endless joy and delight and the realization that your skin — your largest organ and your "living hide," so to speak — is not just an inert covering but a beautiful and faithful friend that, with nurturing and pampering, will reward you with a lifetime of comfort and radiance.

—Stephanie

THE HIGH PRICE OF VANITY

Many of the synthetic chemicals and artificial fragrances in our daily applications of body care products have names that might sound like Greek to us — and because our skin may absorb up to 60 percent of them, they can all be potentially harmful. Once they are in our bodies, our fatty tissue can store many of these chemicals, leading to a host of possible problems. The solution to avoiding these chemicals? Read the label!

Parabens are chemical preservatives found in many body care products. They mimic the hormone estrogen. Many people suffer from allergies or sensitivities to parabens and break out in a rash after applying a paraben-containing product. In fact, some topical parabens have even been detected in human breast tumors.

Other preservatives such as dimethylol dimethyl (DMDM) hydantoin, imidazolidinyl urea, and quaternium-15 are very common and can release trace amounts of formaldehyde into the skin, potentially leading to joint pain and contact dermatitis.

The chemical triethanolamine (TEA), often used as an emulsifier and in cosmetics to adjust pH, may cause allergic reactions, skin and hair dryness, and eye irritation.

Artificial fragrances are often manufactured from petrochemicals and can irritate the skin and strip it of its natural protection. They can even lead to difficulties such as headaches and asthmatic complications.

Synthetic colors such as FD&C or D&C (F = food, D = drugs, and C = cosmetics) followed by a number can be carcinogenic: Red 40, Yellow 5, Yellow 6, and Red 3 are some common examples. Fortunately, many commercial products do use natural coloring agents.

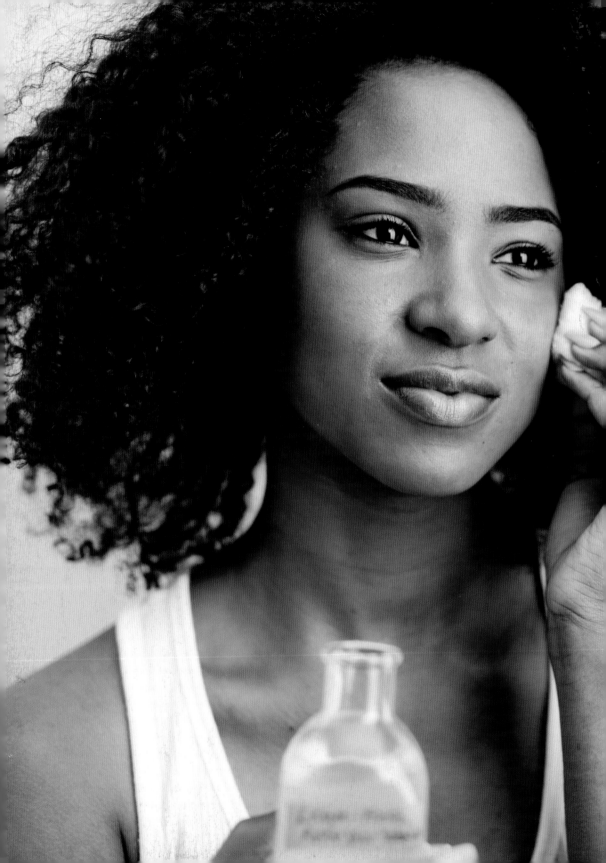

Part One

ACHIEVING BEAUTIFUL SKIN, *Naturally*

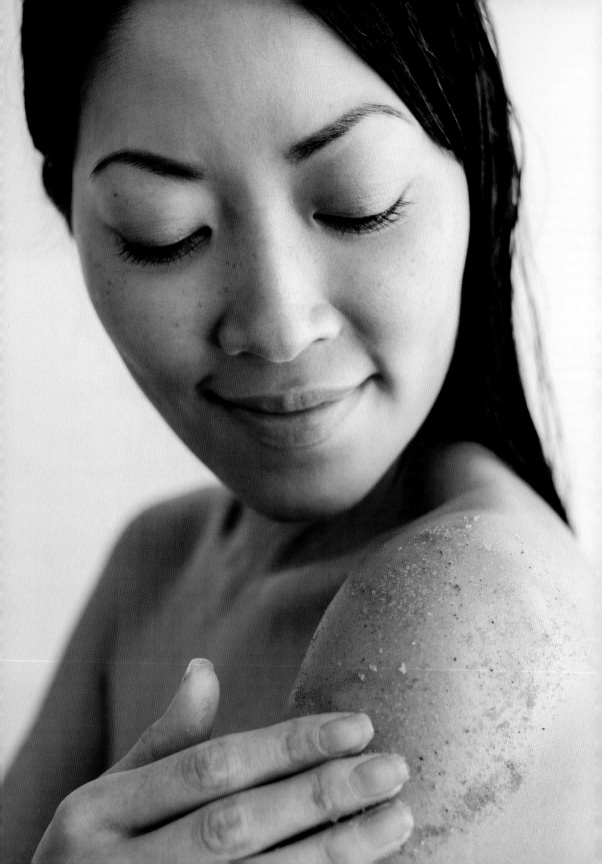

Chapter 1

CARING
FOR YOUR
SKIN

To care properly for your skin, it's important to understand something about its structure and purpose. Knowing how, why, and when to care for your skin and identifying the best formulas for its needs will allow you to keep your skin healthy and beautiful regardless of the climate you live in or your chronological age.

YOUR SKIN

Think of your skin as a beautiful satin robe that you wear night and day. It presents your external beauty and health to the world and at the same time protects your inner being. The skin, or integumentary system, is an actual living system that also includes the hair and nails, various glands, and several specialized receptors. As a complex structure, it performs many essential jobs for the body:

Protects us from physical, chemical, biological, thermal, and electrical damage

Helps the body maintain a steady temperature

Acts as a moisture regulator, preventing excessive entry and evaporation of water

Serves as part of our immune system

Converts ultraviolet rays into vitamin D$_3$, part of the vitamin D complex that helps us maintain strong bones by enhancing the absorption of calcium and other minerals

Serves as a highly sensitive sensory organ, responding to heat, cold, pain, pleasure, and pressure

Stores essential body fat

Secretes sebum, an oily lubricating substance

Assists in detoxification via sweating, which helps the body excrete salts, urea, and toxins

As a general rule, your skin is designed to keep out more things than it lets in. Bacteria can enter through follicular openings, contributing to pimples, boils, folliculitis, and acne, as well as through breaks in or damage to the skin — such as burns, cuts, abrasions, punctures, and ulcers — leading to infections. Its follicular openings and sweat pores also allow many topically applied substances to be absorbed.

Your skin constantly transmits and receives information. If something is amiss, it displays signs of interior or exterior distress. If all is well, it displays radiance.

The skin is our largest body organ; it consists of tissues structurally joined together to perform specific activities. It varies in thickness: the skin on the eyelids is the thinnest — thinner even than the paper these words are printed on — and the skin on the soles of your feet and your palms is the thickest. The skin of an average-size adult weighs approximately 5 to 8 pounds.

Your skin constantly transmits and receives information. If something is amiss, it displays signs of interior or exterior distress. If all is well, it displays radiance.

A Look beneath the Skin

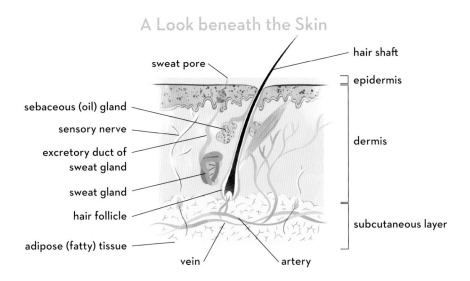

hair shaft

sweat pore

epidermis

sebaceous (oil) gland

sensory nerve

dermis

excretory duct of
sweat gland

sweat gland

hair follicle

subcutaneous layer

adipose (fatty) tissue

vein

artery

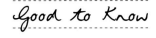

Good to Know

SKINFORMATION

The complex structures of the skin contained within 1 square inch include the following:

- 65 hairs

- 9,500,000 cells

- 95 to 100 sebaceous (oil) glands

- 650 sweat glands

- 19 yards of blood vessels

- 78 yards of nerves

- 78 sensory apparatuses for perceiving heat

- 19,500 sensory cells at the ends of nerve fibers

- 1,300 nerve endings to register pain

- 160 to 165 pressure apparatuses for perceiving touch

- 13 sensory apparatuses for perceiving cold

Adapted from Joel Gerson, *Milady's Standard Textbook for Professional Estheticians*, 8th Edition.

The skin, technically called the *cutis*, has three layers: the epidermal, the dermal, and the subcutaneous. The epidermal layer, or *epidermis*, is the outermost, thinnest layer. Though it contains no blood vessels, it does have many small nerve endings and shows the world your wrinkles, breakouts, dry flakes, laugh lines, sunburns, blisters, age spots, and freckles — in other words, the results of genetics and lifestyle habits, good and bad.

The epidermis consists of a form of soft *keratin* proteins (hair, fingernails, and toenails are made of hard keratin) that are resistant to water and many chemicals and provide a shield of protection from the outside world. It also contains *melanocytes*, the cells that produce your skin's particular pigment.

The dermal layer, or *dermis*, lies just below the epidermis and is a tough, strong, elastic layer of connective tissue. It, along with other connective tissues, secures your internal organs, bones, fluids, and so forth. Its abundant blood supply puts roses in your cheeks and gives you a look of vitality.

Collagen and elastin are two major types of protein fibers found in the dermis. Collagen helps give skin its form and strength. Elastin gives skin its flexibility. Studies show that as we age, collagen production slows and elastin weakens. As a result, skin becomes slack and wrinkles begin to form. Wrinkles are a natural part of the aging process, whether we like it or not. With good care of the skin, we can moderate the effects of aging. But harsh or abrasive skin care products, poor nutrition, lack of hydration, insufficient exercise, and excessive exposure to sun, salt, wind, pollution, and dry air take a toll and can cause the skin to age prematurely. Certain prescription medications and emotional stressors that trigger biochemical responses can also lead to dry, irritated, sensitive skin.

The subcutaneous layer, or *subcutis*, is the layer of adipose, or fatty, tissue that lies beneath the dermis and connects to the underlying muscle tissue. Circulation is maintained here by a network of arteries and lymphatics. A little fat is a good thing as far as your skin is concerned. It keeps your face from looking drawn and hollow and gives your body beautiful contours and smoothness. It provides a strong foundation for your skin and acts as a shock absorber and insulator, protecting your internal organs. And this fat provides your entire body with a storehouse of vital long-term energy reserves to draw upon as necessary. As you age (or crash-diet), the subcutis becomes thinner, leaving behind sagging, unsupported skin.

Achieving Beautiful Skin, Naturally

YOUR NAILS: THE TOUGHEST KIND OF SKIN

Fingernails and toenails, like hair, are appendages of the skin. A nail, or *onyx*, is composed of the hardest keratin. The average growth rate of an adult fingernail is approximately ⅛ inch per month; toenails grow more slowly.

The *cuticle* is the small flap of skin that often hangs over the nail plate, protecting the delicate matrix below. Cuticles can become damaged due to overexposure to water, dry conditions, the application of artificial nails, and contact with detergents, dirt, and chemicals. If a cuticle is damaged, the once-watertight space under the *nail fold* (the deep fold of skin at the base of the nail, where the nail root is embedded) becomes susceptible to moisture and thus a potential breeding ground for bacteria and yeast.

To protect your nails and cuticles, treat them kindly and wear appropriate gloves when necessary. If your cuticles do get dry and ragged, regular therapeutic soaking and moisturizing will revive them. Never cut your cuticles or even push them back vigorously, no matter how ragged they are; you will only damage them further.

If you frequently suffer from cold fingertips, your nails may need extra stimulation to encourage proper blood flow. A daily nail massage with a good oil blend or a weekly at-home buffing can help. If your budget allows, a weekly professional manicure, complete with hand massage, is an indulgence to enjoy. Skip the polish if you wish. In no time, you'll see 10 nails (and cuticles) in beautiful, tip-top condition. A weekly hand reflexology session will also improve circulation to your hands and forearms while simultaneously deeply relaxing your body and mind!

Your nails, like your skin, are mirrors of your general state of health or lifestyle. A healthy nail is smooth or very finely ridged, softly glossy, and translucent pink. Nail disorders such as deep ridges or furrows, thickening, discoloration, dimples, or slow growth can indicate systemic problems like malnutrition or illness or excessive contact with dry air, water, soap, or chemicals. Even tools of the nail technician's trade — polishes, removers, artificial nails, nippers, scissors, brushes, and orangewood sticks — can, if improperly used or unsanitary, physically harm nails or transmit bacteria and fungi.

Parts of the Fingernail

free edge →
nail plate —
lunula —
cuticle —
— nail bed
— nail fold
— matrix

SEVEN KEYS TO VIBRANT SKIN

Your skin, like all the other organs of the body, receives nourishment via blood, which means that your skin is alive. In order to keep your skin, hair, and nails looking their best and running at peak performance, then, you need to give them what they need to survive and thrive.

Follow my seven lifestyle keys to ensure a lifetime of healthy, vibrant good looks and an energetic body:

Daily cleansing

Maximal nutrition intake

Regular consumption of pure water

Regular internal and external detoxification

Daily movement

Moderate exposure to sunlight

Sound sleep

1. Cleanse Your Skin Daily

Because your skin is constantly excreting wastes and shedding dead skin debris (sounds awful, but it's true), daily cleansing is a beauty must. All that's required is a mild, natural cleanser designed for your skin type (see Determining Your Skin Type on page 22). If you wear foundation, powder, blush, or waterproof face and eye makeup, it's absolutely imperative that you remove this layer before going to sleep in order to avoid the possibility of clogged pores, blocked tear ducts, and the formation of blackheads and potential acne. Even if you don't wear makeup, it's a good idea to wash your face prior to bedtime, as the natural sebum on the surface of your skin attracts atmospheric pollutants and dirt like a magnet.

If you perspire a great deal, rinse off and massage your body with a coarse towel, then use a body brush (page 17) or loofah before retiring to remove salt and dead-skin buildup.

2. Maximize Your Nutrition

What you eat directly affects how you look and feel. The quickest and least expensive way to change your looks and feel better mentally and physically is to clean up your diet. You can make effective improvements easily.

According to the US Department of Agriculture, more than two-thirds of adults and one-third of children in the United States are overweight or obese. Studies show that more than 60 percent of our daily calories come from highly processed foods like refined breads, refined grain-based desserts like cookies, and sports drinks, sodas, and juice. As a culture, we love pizza, burgers, fried foods, chips, sugary snacks, and other foods that provide plenty of calories but little nutrition. Studies show that fruits and vegetables make up just 12 percent of the average American diet — and half of that comes from potatoes (chips, fries) and tomatoes (ketchup, pizza sauce, pasta sauce).

As a result, we are often overfed and undernourished. We look and feel older than our years, and we suffer from low energy and vitality and a variety of aches, pains, and illnesses.

Many of the foods you can find in grocery stores today are made with an eye toward corporate profits rather than your maximum fuel potential. Intensive farming practices and poor soil management produce foods that tend to lack taste and nutrients. Add synthetic fertilizers, pesticides, herbicides, and genetic engineering to the mix, and you've got additional woes.

A wholesome, balanced diet nourishes the inner body and is reflected on the outside.

Your diet should consist of foods that are high in complex carbohydrates, high in fiber, moderate in healthy fats, and moderate in lean protein. You should consume daily a wide variety of foods in their whole, natural, preferably organic state, including several servings each of fresh fruits, vegetables, whole grains (as your body tolerates), and beans; a few tablespoons of raw nuts and seeds; and a little extra-virgin olive oil, flaxseed oil, or unrefined coconut oil.

If you eat eggs, look for those that come from certified organically raised chickens. Enjoy them several times a week or even on a daily basis if you avoid other sources of animal protein.

Meat, poultry, and seafood eaters should limit their consumption to 3 to 4 ounces per day (a serving about the size of a deck of cards) and try to buy only organic, free-range chicken or turkey; wild-caught deep-sea fish (such as salmon, cod, mackerel, and haddock) and shellfish; and grass-fed beef or pork from cows and pigs raised without antibiotics and steroids or other hormones. Alternative animal sources of protein such as lamb, venison, goat, and buffalo are another option and are usually untainted by chemicals. Avoid excess consumption of animal proteins; they're often high in fat and totally void of fiber.

You can also fulfill your protein needs with vegetarian choices such as organic soybean products (tofu, tempeh, and edamame), grain/veggie burgers, rice and pea protein powders, nut butters, seeds, sprouted breads, bean sprouts, seaweed, and bean and grain combinations.

A wholesome, balanced diet nourishes the inner body and is reflected on the outside.

WHOLE-FOOD SUPPLEMENTS

Along with a whole-foods diet, nutritional supplements also have their benefits for your well-being. No matter how balanced you think your diet is, it could be lacking in one nutrient or another. Supplements help fill in the nutritional gaps so that you look and feel your best.

I believe that the most effective supplements are derived from whole, real foods (as opposed to being entirely synthetic). I take my three favorite supplements daily. Combined, they contain all of the specific nutrients that help support healthy aging, promote well-being, and nourish skin, hair, and nails.

Green drink blend. Nearly every morning, I toss a handful of frozen raspberries, strawberries, mango chunks, or banana chunks into the blender, then add a cup or more of homemade almond milk, a dollop of plain goat's milk yogurt, a scoop of pea protein blend, and 2 tablespoons of an organic green plant powder. The one I use contains "powerhouse plants" including chlorella, spirulina, barley grass, wheat grass, and alfalfa.

When choosing a green plant powder, make sure the product label states that the ingredients were organically grown and processed immediately after being harvested to preserve the enzymes and vitamins they contain. The grasses taste the way a freshly mowed lawn smells — sweet and green. The blend I use, like many others, is also available in easy-to-swallow capsules.

OPCs (oligomeric proanthocyanidins). Yup, it's a tongue twister, but here's a short explanation: OPCs are recognized as one of the most potent categories of antioxidants, which help slow the effects of aging or, as some might say, serve as powerful "youthifying agents." They fight the free radicals that cause *oxidation*, the process responsible for the rusting of metal, the browning of a cut apple, or the appearance of premature wrinkling and brown age spots on your body. OPCs are present only in plants and have blue-green, yellow, red, and purple pigments.

You can find OPC supplements in liquid or powdered form at any good health food store. They are often derived from purple and red grapes, prunes, raisins, blueberries, blackberries, red bilberries, lingonberries, raspberries, spinach, kale, currants, rose hips, turmeric, ginger, pine bark, grape seeds, green tea, ginkgo leaf, hawthorn leaf, and oregano. In fact, I recommend that you include many of these foods in your daily diet. An added bonus: liquid OPC formulations are usually quite delicious, tasting like fruit juice.

Raw sunflower seeds, pumpkin seeds, and walnuts. Mix equal parts of raw sunflower seeds, raw pumpkin seeds, and walnuts. Carry a bag of this tasty, crunchy treat with you as a healthy fast-food snack, or toss a handful in your daily salad in lieu of croutons. For a zestier taste, sprinkle a bit of sea salt or your favorite herb seasoning over the mix.

These raw seeds and nuts contain essential dietary fats, including vitamin E and omega-3s, plus substantial amounts of iron, selenium, manganese, copper, and zinc, and may be some of the most powerful munchies in the anti-wrinkle arsenal. Fat preserves your skin's suppleness and youthful sheen. Raw fats also have potent anti-inflammatory properties, promoting heart health and pain relief.

Another option: consume a tablespoon or two of fresh flaxseed oil, superior quality extra-virgin olive oil, fish oil derived from anchovies, sardines, and mackerel, or unrefined coconut oil. Consume different oils each day to ensure that you receive a variety of essential fatty acids.

3. Drink Water — the Elixir of Youth and Health

What's the difference between a plum and a prune, an ocean marsh and the Sahara Desert, and the smooth skin of a teenager and the sagging and wrinkled skin of a 90-year-old? Water — the simple, pure essence of life that makes up approximately 70 percent of each of us. It's one of the most important and most abundant inorganic

Tips
GOOD FOOD AND GOOD LOOKS: MAKE THE CONNECTION

Carol Alt was one of the fashion world's first official supermodels, having been featured in hundreds of magazines and ad campaigns since the 1980s. She's also an accomplished actress and author of *Eating in the Raw*, an eye-opening treatise on the role a raw-food diet can play in lifelong health and good looks.

As a raw foodist, Alt believes in eating only foods that have not been cooked or chemically altered by heat, which can destroy many heat-sensitive vitamins and alter the protein structure of animal products. The raw-food diet includes fruit and vegetable salads, juices, smoothies, nuts, seeds, sprouts, raw dairy, sushi, raw shellfish, and steak tartar. According to Alt, consuming a completely raw diet has done a world of good for her overall health, skin quality, and vitality — all of which make her look much younger than her years.

While a 100 percent raw diet is not for everyone, eating this way from time to time can make you feel great. Regardless of whether you are a raw-food purist or not, a raw-food diet features many important elements that should be incorporated into your daily nutrition: large quantities of fresh, raw, preferably organic fruits and vegetables, sprouted grains, and nuts and seeds. These will go a long way toward improving the way you look *and* feel.

substances in the human body. In fact, it is by far the most abundant material in all tissues, with the exception of tooth enamel and bone. Your blood, the "living highway," is primarily composed of water.

The body literally can't move or function, inside or out, without water. You can't bend or stretch, blink, yawn, smile, jump up and down, poop, breathe, sweat, or even think without water lubricating every part of your physical being or assisting with the transport of nutrients, oxygen, and other vital substances.

You also cannot be beautiful, energetic, and healthy without sufficient water intake. With ample moisture, the elastin and collagen matrix in the dermis layer of your skin stays plump. Conversely, a dehydrated person ages prematurely and is exhausted.

Try to consume at least six glasses of water a day for optimal well-being. If you hate drinking plain water, try adding a squeeze of lime, lemon, or orange to the glass. A splash of cranberry or cherry juice concentrate added to water also makes a deliciously tangy treat. Or drink the juice of raw whole fruits and veggies (not canned or pasteurized juice), which contains vital nutrients as well as water.

4. Detoxify, Inside and Out

Simply stated, your skin serves as the interface between your inner and outer worlds. To keep both worlds functioning well and feeling comfortable, regular removal of bodily wastes must take place via natural

---

Good to Know

TESTING YOUR SKIN'S AGE

Want to know your skin's biological age? Pinch the skin on the back of your hand, hold for a few seconds, and then release it. If you're under 30 years of age, the skin will quickly return to its original contour. If you are between 30 and 50, you can often begin to see the skin stand up for a second or two before recovering. At age 50 and beyond, the skin may stand up for a number of seconds, a sign that its support network has been altered or that the body as a whole is undergoing changes that are visible at the skin's surface.

There are variables to this timetable, of course, depending on your diet, fluid intake, and lifestyle habits and the degree of environmental damage that your skin has suffered over the years. I've seen 35-year-old skin that looks and acts more like 55 due to decades of smoking, neglect, and poor lifestyle and dietary habits. On the flip side, I've seen clients older than 60 with plump, nearly wrinkle-free skin, a reflection of regular nurturing and care of their skin and body — inside and out.

internal elimination channels and the routine removal of deposits such as sweat, sebum, and dead skin cell buildup from the top layer of your skin.

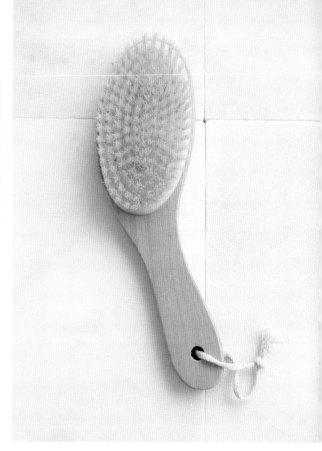

Body brush with natural-fiber bristles.

INTERNAL FLUSHING: FIBER AND WATER

What goes in must come out. Ample fluid intake combined with a fiber-filled diet keeps the digestive system moving right along, eliminating toxins via your colon and preventing them from surfacing on your skin as rashes and blemishes. Impurities that aren't disposed of in a timely manner via the kidneys, bladder, liver, lungs, and large intestine will find an alternative exit — which is why the skin is sometimes referred to as the "third kidney." Staying "regular" contributes to physical comfort, does a world of good for your mood, and keeps your skin clear and radiant.

EXTERNAL BRUSHING: BEAUTY AND THE BODY BRUSH

One of my favorite health-promoting rituals, which I enjoy nearly every morning, is body brushing (sometimes called *dry brushing* because it's performed on dry skin).

Body brushing — an age-old tradition undergoing a renaissance in today's wellness spas — takes only about 5 minutes, and you do it before showering or bathing. It stimulates the sebaceous glands, thereby encouraging natural lubrication of your skin; removes the top layer of dead skin cells, leading to significant exfoliation and skin that's polished and silky; improves circulation and increases blood flow to the surface of the body; and activates the entire lymphatic system, thereby aiding in natural detoxification.

Another benefit that I've noticed from body brushing is improved tone in the "jiggle-prone" parts of my body like my upper arms and inner thighs. In addition, my complexion is rosier, body lotions and oils penetrate more easily, and — a bonus I didn't expect — it doesn't take me 30 minutes to wake up in the morning, like it used to! For me, body brushing is equivalent to a shot of espresso. Not bad for a 5-minute beauty treatment!

Perform this treatment daily. Here's how:

Using a medium-soft natural-fiber brush that's designed specifically for use on the body (the bristle area being roughly the size of your palm and preferably with a handle), simply brush your entire body — don't skip any areas except your face and genitals (and breasts, if you're a woman) — for 5 minutes or so, depending on your body size. Do not brush hard. You'll have to start very gently at first (even more so if you have very sensitive skin) and work your way up to more vigorous brushing. Never scrub, however; your skin is not the tub!

Brush in the direction of your heart as much as possible. Begin by brushing your hands, including the area in between the fingers, then work upward to your arms, underarms, neck, chest, and upper back. Next, brush each leg, beginning with the feet and working upward toward the groin, buttocks, lower back, and sides. End at your stomach, using a counterclockwise spiral motion to brush this area.

As a final step, jump in the tub or shower and bathe as usual. All of the dead skin you just loosened will be washed away. Afterward, be sure to pat — not rub — your skin until it's almost dry, and then apply your favorite body oil or moisturizer.

Your skin may take a while to get used to body brushing, but soon enough you'll find that it makes you feel wonderfully invigorated, and your skin will glow. If you're just beginning, your skin may be a bit red immediately afterward, but as it adjusts and becomes firmer, that redness should ease back to only a pinkish tinge (depending on your pigmentation) that lasts for about 5 minutes, until your circulation calms. If your skin remains red or pink for a longer period, then either the brush bristles are too firm or you're brushing too hard.

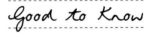

Good to Know

WHY IT WORKS

Over the course of an average day your skin eliminates more than a pound of waste, including perspiration. In fact, about one-third of all the body's impurities are excreted through the skin. If your skin is not carrying out normal elimination due to poor hygiene, illness, dry skin buildup, medication side effects, nutritional deficiencies, or repeated applications of mineral oil–based, pore-clogging body lotions or waterproof synthetic chemical sunscreens, then your kidneys, large intestine, liver, and lungs may become overwhelmed and begin to operate on a subpar level. Anything you can do to improve skin function improves the function of the other organs of elimination.

Achieving Beautiful Skin, Naturally

It's a good idea to wash your body brush with mild soap and water every week or so to keep it free of odor and skin debris.

Note: Avoid dry brushing altogether if your skin is sunburned, windburned, rashy, or otherwise irritated.

5. Keep Moving to Look and Feel Your Best

Lead your body in the right direction, and the health of the skin follows. Regular physical exercise boosts lymphatic flow and circulation, improves digestion, stimulates your metabolic fire and the process of waste removal from the internal organs and skin, and delivers a surge of oxygen to your body, invigorating every organ and allowing your skin to take on radiance. In circulating nutrient-rich blood and oxygen, the body prioritizes the internal organs; without the circulatory boost that regular exercise provides, your extremities, including your skin, hair, and nails, will not receive all the fortification that they could, and your skin will not manifest optimal health and beauty.

Daily exercise is also vital to your emotional well-being. It can energize you in the morning or help you unwind after work, eliminating or reducing the stresses of the day. Exercise acts as a natural antidepressant.

Try to exercise in the fresh air and sunshine as often as possible and vigorously enough so that you work up a good sweat. Sweating cools your skin and eliminates waste through your pores. Choose whatever activity you enjoy: walking, biking, jogging, swimming, Pilates, yoga, tai chi, aerobics classes, tennis, or even skating. If you have a garden plot and like to grow fresh veggies, gardening is a great way to stretch and strengthen your body — plus you'll have a bounty of fresh, nourishing foods as your reward! There really is an activity for everyone. It's up to you to find it and stick with it, or to choose several and alternate to keep things interesting!

6. Give Yourself Some Exposure: A Little Sun Is a Good Thing

We've become a sun-phobic society. Yet most living things — plants, animals, and people — need at least a little sunshine in order to survive and thrive. Certainly, *overexposure* to the sun is the single most damaging factor to your skin. It's not just sunburns but also suntans (and the associated skin dehydration) that represent damage to your skin, and that damage is cumulative over a lifetime.

Yet sunshine feels good on your skin and helps your body absorb calcium by causing your skin to produce that part of the vitamin D complex that strengthens bones. Sun exposure helps reduce stress and blood pressure, balances hormone levels, increases the body's production of feel-good serotonin, and aids in healing eczema, acne, psoriasis, and poison plant rashes.

Approximately 30 to 45 minutes of daily unprotected exposure to sunlight can help preserve your sanity and the health of your bones and skin. To avoid skin damage, try to get that sunshine early in the morning (before 10 A.M.) or late in the day (after 4 P.M.). If you live in the north, where sunshine is sometimes limited in the winter and temperatures can be quite cold, try to expose your face and hands for at least 15 minutes daily. Many health professionals have observed a rise in the occurrence of osteoporosis, spontaneous fractures of the small bones of the feet, vitamin D deficiencies, skin diseases, mood imbalances, and seasonal affective disorder around the globe because our lives are increasingly sedentary and spent indoors, with long car commutes between work and home. Getting adequate sun exposure can positively affect the incidence of these conditions.

Sun exposure helps reduce stress and blood pressure, balances hormone levels, increases the body's production of feel-good serotonin, and aids in healing eczema, acne, psoriasis, and poison plant rashes.

Sun exposure is a subject of much debate, however, and if your health professional or dermatologist has advised you to avoid the sun at all costs due to various health concerns, then your body will require other sources of vitamin D. This essential nutrient can be found in egg yolks, cod liver oil, cold-water fish oils, vitamin D_3–supplemented animal or vegan milks, organ meats, salmon, sardines, and herring.

While brief periods of unprotected sun exposure may be beneficial, when you intend to spend a longer period of time in the sun, it's important to apply a natural, nontoxic sunscreen prior to exposure, wear

protective clothing, and use common sun sense: don't stay in the sun for hours on end with no protection of any kind or without reapplying sunscreen regularly, and avoid exposure during the middle of the day, when the sun's rays are at their strongest. These strategies will help prevent premature aging, uneven skin tone and blotching, and exposure that may cause skin cancer.

Though it's important to wear sunscreen, the synthetic chemicals in most commercial products can be irritating, especially for people who exercise outdoors. Sunscreens can sting if they drip into your eyes or nose and can cause skin rashes when their chemical base mixes with sweat. Natural sunscreens, such as those containing titanium dioxide and zinc oxide, provide a physical sun-reflective barrier, offer a relatively high SPF, and greatly reduce or eliminate irritation. Natural oil blends containing jojoba or sesame oil are beneficial skin emollients and conditioners that also provide a natural low SPF. See chapter 6 for some natural sunscreen recipes.

As for tanning, if you *must* have a deep sun-kissed hue, then try a good-quality natural self-tanning lotion or cream. Follow the directions to the letter, make sure you exfoliate prior to application, and take the time to apply an even layer. The results are quite realistic if the lotion is applied correctly.

Observing common sun sense beginning in your early teen years can virtually stop the visible aging clock. But at any age, it's never too late to begin to care for your skin and health in the sun.

COMMON SUN SENSE
Tips

Many years ago, after one of my best friends and I completed an exhausting 5-mile power walk through the baking-hot Texas hill country (slathered in natural sunscreen, of course), we laughed at how bedraggled and red-faced we looked. My friend then reminded me of this bit of wisdom often attributed to Hunter S. Thompson: "Life should not be a journey to the grave with the intention of arriving safely in a pretty and well-preserved body, but rather to skid in broadside in a cloud of smoke, thoroughly used up, totally worn out, and loudly proclaiming, 'Wow! What a ride!'"

After walking in the south Texas heat, that's exactly how we both felt: used up, covered in sweat, and totally worn out — but also happy, relaxed, and stress-free. By far the most important accomplishment of our walk, though, was catching up on the important gossip of the week! Exercising with a friend is a terrific time for socializing.

Outdoor exercise and sports can be fun, and at times even exhilarating, but it doesn't have to come at the expense of your skin's health. If you're an avid outdoorswoman or outdoorsman, keep Mother Nature's sun, heat, salt, drying wind, cold, or arid climate at bay by always drinking plenty of water and wearing a shield of moisturizers, natural sunscreens, protective clothing, and sunglasses!

7. Seek Deep, Restful Sleep

Did you get a good night's sleep last night? For many people, the answer is no. Sleep is often the first thing we sacrifice due to work commitments, children's demands, lifestyle choices, or the activity of today's hustle-and-bustle world. In fact, sleep doesn't get much attention until it's sorely missing. The solution: instead of thinking of sleep as a luxury or as something you can put off and catch up on later, think of it as an essential nutrient, just like vitamin C or water. Nighttime is the right time for renewal, and those prized hours when you sleep are the optimal time for your body's repair and rejuvenation.

Your body produces human growth hormone, which aids in the repair of damaged cells, including those of the skin, hair, and nails, while you sleep. When you're sleep-deprived, your body struggles to maintain itself mentally and physically. Lack of sleep shows up as dark circles or puffy skin under your eyes, haggard and sallow skin, dull hair, lackluster nails, low energy, weakened immunity, mental meltdowns, depression, irregular appetite, and lack of sexual interest. Sleep deprivation can also trigger the release of cortisol, your stress hormone. Overproduction of cortisol ages your skin and contributes to unmistakable signs of fatigue (plus it stimulates weight gain around your midsection). You can't put your best face forward when you're running on empty!

We call a solid night of shut-eye our *beauty sleep* or *beauty rest* because it's one of the best (and least expensive) beauty secrets of models and celebrities or anyone who depends on physical appearance for his or her livelihood. You can spend scads of money on the latest eye cream or trendy spa treatments, but a good dose of sleep is the most effective beauty booster of all — and even more important, it's the foundation of your overall well-being.

DETERMINING YOUR SKIN TYPE

Accurately assessing and caring for your skin type is key to having skin that is irresistible to touch and behold. Too many people treat their skin with the wrong products, and consequently, instead of improving its condition, they worsen it. What's more, skin type can change with the seasons, personal environment, health, and lifestyle. Yours may be different today than it was even a few months ago. It's important to know your current skin type in order to care for your skin in the best way.

Your skin probably falls into one of the following skin type categories, though some people may overlap two categories. Whether you lie in one classification or bridge two, it's important to assess your skin honestly and without judgment.

In each category you'll find ingredient and formula suggestions for recipes and methods of care. If you run across a particular ingredient or term that you don't understand, please see the index at the back of this book for all page references to that item. You'll be able to find an explanation or a formula recipe in no time. Also note that in the glossary (page 206), you'll find descriptions and explanations for all the ingredients used in the recipes in this book.

Normal or Balanced Skin

This skin is neither too oily nor too dry. It's usually free of blemishes but may form blackheads. It may get a little oily in the T-zone (the forehead, nose, and chin area) or in the upper-back region 4 to 6 hours after cleansing, depending on humidity and temperature. The pores are normal in size. The entire body may suffer from surface dehydration in very cold weather. Normal skin is a balanced skin functioning as it should and is everyone's desired type.

When you improve your appearance, you also boost your morale. And we all function better and are more comfortable when we know we have presented our best to our critical selves and to the world.

Virginia Castleton,
The Handbook of Natural Beauty

CARE RECOMMENDATIONS

Use a mild soap as a cleanser *if you must* (see On My Soapbox, page 32), but it's best to use a gentle, water-based, nonfoaming cleanser or a lotion-type or creamy cleanser on both your face and body. Finely ground oat, nut, or seed blends and clay blends are simple nourishing cleansers as well. Follow facial cleansing with an application of an herbal hydrosol mist or an herbal vinegar or tea toner to refresh and further cleanse the skin. Lavender, rose, calendula, lady's mantle, German chamomile, and rosemary are great mild herb choices. The moisturizer you choose for both your face and body should be a lightweight yet protective lotion designed to enhance and seal in moisture. An herbal elixir or facial oil is a conditioning, lubricating, and protective option for the face. If your skin is prone to a bit of oiliness, avoid anything too heavy.

SPECIAL INTENSIVE THERAPIES

For the face, use a weekly moisturizing mask or pore-refining, oil-absorbing clay mask. You can decide which treatment will best benefit your skin in any particular week — remember that skin condition fluctuates! These masks can be used on the chest, upper back, and throat as well. Fruit-acid masks made from papaya, apple, pineapple, or raspberry pulp are best used once or twice weekly to gently exfoliate, minimize fine lines, and smooth the skin. A weekly herbal facial steam will help keep pores clean.

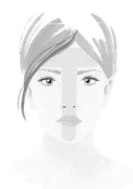

T-zone

Selected Recipes for Normal Skin

Oily Skin

This skin has medium to large pores in the T-zone area and perhaps on the cheeks, shoulders, neck, chest, and back. Overactive sebaceous glands can give oily skin a shiny appearance within an hour after cleansing. This skin oftentimes has clogged pores and may be prone to mild, moderate, or weeping/active acne, which is highly inflamed with open pustules. Makeup seems to disappear or "slide off" oily skin after a few hours. Heat and humidity tend to increase its sebum production, whereas cooler temperatures and lower humidity are a boon for an oily complexion. Surface dehydration may occur in very cold, dry weather. A bonus: because it is well lubricated, oily skin is not prone to fine lines and wrinkles and tends to reveal its true age quite slowly.

CARE RECOMMENDATIONS

For your face and body you can use a gentle bar or liquid soap, such as a castile soap designed for infants or a soap made from goat's milk, olive oil, or vegetable glycerin, but it's best to use a water-based gel or lotion-type cleanser specifically formulated for oily skin, a finely ground cleanser (oat, nut, or seed), or a clay-blend cleanser that does not dry out the skin's surface. Facial skin should be cleansed twice daily. If oily skin becomes dehydrated on the surface, it will tend to produce more oil to compensate, which is not what you want. Your goal is to remove excess oil without stripping the skin of its protective barrier. Learn to equate "squeaky clean" with "dried out."

Selected Recipes for Oily Skin

Classic Rosewater and Glycerin Freshening Cleanser, page 67

Refreshing Skin Wash, page 70

Lemony Whip Cleansing Cream, page 78

Refreshing Astringent, page 83

Acne-Soothing Astringent, page 88

Tranquility Toner, page 94

Thyme to Heal Tonic, page 98

Green Goddess Purifying Clay Mask, page 104

Rosy Red Balancing Clay Mask, page 106

Outta Here, Oil! Skin Scrub, page 139

Light and Lively Moisturizer, page 155

Out, Damn Spot! Antiblemish Elixir, page 165

Healing Thyme Elixir, page 166

Follow facial cleansing with the application of a gentle herbal vinegar or tea toner made with astringent herbs such as yarrow, sage, lemon balm, thyme, lemongrass, rosemary, parsley, or peppermint in order to remove cleanser residue and reestablish a proper pH level. If you also suffer from an oily body, make enough Balance Restorer (page 87) to use as a finishing rinse before you get out of the shower. An application of commercially prepared aloe vera juice following your bath or shower is always beneficial for oily skin. Feel free to apply your choice of an oil-moderating liquid to your face and body as often as necessary throughout the day. This procedure will remove excess sebum but will not dry your skin.

Depending on the degree of your skin's oiliness, a moisturizer may not be necessary for your face or body. A light, hydrating herbal hydrosol mist such as lemon balm, rose geranium, rosemary, or rose may be enough to keep your facial skin moist throughout the day. You can apply a light moisturizing lotion to your body as needed. For the face, you can use an herbal elixir or facial oil specially formulated for oily skin to help normalize sebum production.

SPECIAL INTENSIVE THERAPIES
Use a clay mask or gentle exfoliating scrub twice a week to discourage the formation of blackheads, reduce the appearance of enlarged pores, and minimize breakouts. Fruit-acid masks used twice a week will remove dead skin cell buildup, refine the skin's surface, and minimize pore size. All masks and scrubs that you use on your face can be used on the body as well.

Note: Do not use a granular scrub of any kind on your face or body if you suffer from acne, eczema, psoriasis, poison plant irritation, or any other type of skin inflammation; scrubs can aggravate these conditions.

A weekly herbal facial steam using sage, rosemary, strawberry leaf, yarrow, peppermint, or other astringent herbs will help detoxify your facial skin and increase circulation. As an overnight spot remedy for minor blemishes or more active pimples, combine a drop of clove, tea tree, thyme, or lavender essential oil with a bit of clay and water to form a paste and dab this directly on the spot to disinfect, absorb oil, and kill bacteria.

Dry Skin

This skin lacks natural oil and moisture, the basic requirements for a healthy glow. It may appear flaky or scaly and feel rough, tight, or dry throughout the day. Dry skin has small pores and feels taut almost immediately after cleansing. It develops lines and wrinkles more rapidly than any other skin type and tends to age prematurely.

Tips
GOT DRY SKIN? MAKE OIL YOUR BEST FRIEND

Here's my lasting solution to very dry body skin in the winter months: body oil. Every day after showering, I roughly towel-dry, leaving my skin slightly damp, and then apply my favorite body oil, massaging it into my skin. I top that off with a layer of body lotion or cream. This double treatment acts as a protective barrier, preventing evaporation of the natural moisture in my skin and locking in the moisture I just received from the shower. This procedure works so well that I rarely have winter-dry, itchy skin anymore!

Dry skin loves warm temperatures and humidity, but the winter can be a real challenge. Cold temperatures and winter air rob the skin of moisture, making it prone to irritation, sensitivity, redness, and chapping.

CARE RECOMMENDATIONS

You must avoid soap on your face and body at all costs. It's much too drying! Instead, use a moisturizing lotion-type cleanser, a creamy cleanser, or a finely ground oat, nut, or seed cleanser.

For toning and hydrating, use a classic rosewater and glycerin blend. Additionally, herbal teas such as German chamomile, calendula, fennel, lavender, lemon balm, marshmallow root, and comfrey root make excellent soothing facial toners. These gentle teas also make good after-bath splashes to hydrate dry and possibly sensitive skin. A quick spritz of chamomile, neroli, or lavender herbal hydrosol mist can alleviate thirsty skin any time of the day.

Good to Know

THE pH FACTOR

You've seen it on everything from shampoos to soaps to toners and creams, but what exactly is pH? It's a measure of the acidity or alkalinity of a substance, on a scale of 0 to 14, with the neutral point being 7. Anything below a 7 on the pH scale is acidic. Anything above a 7 is alkaline. When normal and balanced, your skin is typically mildly acidic, with a pH averaging between 5 and 6.

Most shampoos and especially bar soaps have a pH between 8 and 11, while most toners, astringents, and face splashes have a pH between 4.5 and 6, making them more on the skin-loving acidic side.

Your skin maintains a healthy pH by forming an acid mantle from the combined secretions of your sweat and oil glands. With many cleansers ranging from mild to high degrees of alkalinity, it's important to apply a toner or astringent appropriate for your skin type after cleansing to return your skin to its proper pH. Such products help prevent bacterial penetration as well as the flaking, dryness, and tightness that can come from using soap-based cleansers. Diluted herbal vinegar, lemon water, various herb teas, and hydrosols are ideal mildly acidic solutions for restoring skin pH.

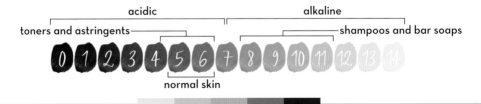

Never forget to moisturize your face and body. Use a rich cream or lotion that provides a barrier against dehydration and keeps moisture in the skin. You can also use an herbal facial elixir or facial oil designed especially for the needs of dry or sensitive skin. In winter, underneath my moisturizer, I use my Repair and Restore Remedy on page 168. Sometimes I apply it again, atop my moisturizer if the weather is severely cold and arid or I'm going to be outside for an extended time. When you've lived through a number of arid, cold, moisture-sapping New England winters, you quickly learn to layer moisturizers, much as you layer clothing — the more layers, the more protection from the biting cold.

Selected Recipes for Dry Skin

SPECIAL INTENSIVE THERAPIES

If you like to bathe in the tub, you can cleanse your body with a small drawstring bath bag filled with ground oats. Once wet, the oatmeal covers your skin with moisturizing and soothing oat milk.

A mucilaginous fennel seed, marshmallow root, or comfrey root facial steam once a week helps hydrate the skin and cleanse the pores. Use a moisturizing mask once or twice a week as needed. For gentle facial exfoliation, try a weekly organic yogurt or fruit-acid mask made from apple or raspberry pulp. At least a couple of times per week, using a light touch, exfoliate your entire body (minus your face) with a fine sugar, sea salt, oat, nut, or seed scrub to remove the buildup of dead skin cells. Gentle exfoliation is necessary to promote the absorption of your moisturizer; otherwise, all of the product's moisture will remain on the surface of the skin and you'll wonder why it's not doing its job. The nightly use of an emollient eye cream or thin application of your favorite base oil will condition the delicate tissue in this area, which is prone to premature wrinkling.

Combination Skin

People with combination skin have two or three skin types on their face. Their skin may be oily through the T-zone, where most of the oil glands are, and normal to dry toward the cheeks and sides of the face. In combination skin, the T-zone generally has enlarged pores and visible blackheads and may be prone to minor breakouts or even acne, while the cheeks and sides of the face and neck may feel normal and balanced or dry and tight, with possible surface flakiness.

This skin type is seasonally aggravated. In winter the oily areas tend to normalize, while the dry areas feel parched. When heat and humidity rise, the T-zone increases its sebum production and the dry areas usually normalize.

CARE RECOMMENDATIONS

Combination skin is frequently sensitive. Always treat it with TLC. Use products that regulate and normalize sebum production for the entire face and upper body. Cleanse with a gentle, water-based, nonfoaming or lotion-type cleanser, though the Ever-So-Gentle Soap-Lover's Face and Body Wash (page 71) may be used by those of you who prefer a gentle sudsing cleanser. Finely ground oat, nut, seed, milk, or clay blends are also nourishing cleansers. With combination skin, the skin of the body — with the exception of the chest and upper back, which are occasionally oily — is usually normal. If you want to use soap as your body cleanser, try a nonirritating clear vegetable glycerin, olive oil, or goat's milk type or a mild liquid castile soap designed for infants.

Selected Recipes for Combination Skin

Refreshing Skin Wash, page 70

Ever-So-Gentle Soap-Lover's Face and Body Wash, page 71

Lemony Whip Cleansing Cream, page 78

Skin-Softening Strawberry Cleanser, page 81

Lemon Refresher, page 84

Grease-Be-Gone Parsley and Peppermint Astringent, page 86

Deep-Cleansing Astringent, page 91

Rosy Red Balancing Clay Mask, page 106

No-More-Pores Double Mask, page 108

Refreshing Pore Cleanser, page 131

Light and Lively Moisturizer, page 155

Cocoa Butter Lotion, page 156

Say Goodnight to Wrinkles Eye Therapy, page 161

Healing Thyme Elixir, page 166

For toning, a mild herbal vinegar infused with German chamomile, lavender, rosemary, fennel, rose, comfrey root, or calendula will help control excess oil and also hydrate dry areas. Any one of these herbs can be made into a tea and applied as a facial toner or used as a body splash immediately after showering or bathing. Rose, lavender, neroli, rosemary, lemon balm, and chamomile hydrosols are great hydrating mists to have on hand during the day to prevent surface dehydration. One of my favorite pore-tightening and skin-softening toner blends for combination skin is a brew made from 2 teaspoons dried yarrow and 1 cup of boiling water. Steep for 15 minutes, strain, and add ½ teaspoon vegetable glycerin. Stir to combine. Keep refrigerated for 1 week, then toss any unused toner and make a new batch.

For conditioning the face, try an herbal elixir or facial oil. Use one designed for oily skin in the warmer months and one for dry skin in the colder months. If you feel the need for more intense moisturizing, apply a light- to medium-weight lotion to the driest areas only. For the body, a light lotion is all you need unless you live or work in an arid environment.

SPECIAL INTENSIVE THERAPIES

Regular exfoliation of the skin on both the face and oilier parts of the body using a non-abrasive mask removes dead skin buildup to keep pores open. Once or twice a week, use a pore-refining clay, yogurt, oatmeal, or fruit-acid mask to improve this skin's texture and minimize pore size. You can also enjoy a facial steam once a week using a mildly astringent herb of your choice, such as lemon balm, peppermint, rosemary, thyme, or lemon peel, to improve the tendency of combination skin toward sluggish circulation.

Sensitive Skin

Environmentally reactive is how I like to refer to skin that is sensitive. It tends to overreact to outside forces such as skin care products, sunlight, and changes in temperature

Tips
PATCH TEST

If you have sensitive skin or are prone to allergies, it's best to test yourself for adverse reactions to the herbs called for in any recipe you're planning to use. To do this, perform a *patch test*: Prepare a paste with ½ teaspoon of the herb in question and a small amount of boiling water, and apply a small portion of the paste to clean skin on the inside of your elbow. Cover with an adhesive bandage and leave on for 12 to 24 hours.

If you're concerned about a potential reaction to an essential oil, dilute 1 or 2 drops with 1 teaspoon of a bland vegetable oil such as sunflower or olive oil, saturate a cotton ball with the mixture, and apply in the same way and in the same general location as the herb paste.

To test any other ingredient, simply apply a small amount to a spot in the same area on your arm and cover with a bandage for the same amount of time.

If any ingredient causes a rash or redness to appear, *do not* use it. You may be able to substitute an ingredient with similar properties; see the Ingredient Dictionary (page 215) for possible substitutes.

and humidity. This skin type easily blushes, sunburns, develops rashes, and becomes irritated. Especially when more mature, it typically displays *couperose* conditions — that is, it's characterized by dilated or expanded capillaries. A diffused redness, or *erythema*, is generally concentrated on the nose, cheeks, and chin. If not treated extremely gently, sensitive skin will simply appear "unhappy" or "unsettled."

Selected Recipes for Sensitive Skin

Crisp, dry winter air can upset sensitive skin, leaving it drier and more prone to irritation. Summer's heat, humidity, and increased exposure to sunlight can also wreak havoc, leading to itchy or blotchy skin, blemishes, and general ruddiness.

CARE RECOMMENDATIONS

Follow all recommendations for dry skin (page 25), unless your skin is normal to oily, in which case use a lightweight to medium-weight moisturizer for both your face and body. Cleanse only with an ultra-soft cloth — no terry towels, facial loofah sponges, or facial brushes on this delicate skin! If you choose to exfoliate your body using a body brush for dry brushing (page 17), please proceed gently, using a rather soft body brush, and *never* scrub your skin.

SPECIAL INTENSIVE THERAPIES

Follow the recommendations for dry skin (page 25). When choosing any product or ingredient, *gentle*, *nonabrasive*, and *fragrance-free* are the key words to look for.

Mature Skin

Skin can generally be considered mature when it loses tone and exhibits a crepe-like texture — that is, it's saggy and loose, with many fine lines and at least a few shallow or even deep wrinkles. People over the age of 50 will eventually develop mature skin as part of the natural aging process, but I've seen prematurely aged skin on individuals as young as their late 30s, and for the lucky few these signs don't reveal themselves until the early 60s. Good genes, plenty of natural oil in the skin, a healthy lifestyle, sound nutrition, and consistent proper skin care all determine when and to what extent mature skin appears.

Mature skin tends to be dry but can be normal or slightly oily in the T-zone, especially if the skin was oily earlier on. If you are over 50 and have oily skin, however, consider it a boon — you'll wrinkle slower and later than your friends. Mature skin is generally more comfortable in warmer climates with higher humidity. In cooler, more arid surroundings, mature skin ages faster and tends to suffer from additional dryness. Such skin may also have hyperpigmentation (age spots, freckles, or liver spots), depending on an individual's history of sun exposure, smoking, and alcohol consumption.

CARE RECOMMENDATIONS

Moisture retention is key to preventing the rapid increase in fine lines and wrinkle depth, so it's important not to use drying soap, especially on the face. Remember that the collagen and elastin matrix within the dermis layer depends on constant hydration to maintain plumpness. For facial cleansing, use a gentle lotion- or cream-type cleanser once or twice a day if you have dry skin or a lighter lotion-type cleanser if your skin is normal to oily. Finely ground oats, almonds, and fat-rich sunflower seeds make super-moisturizing cleansers for the face and body. You could also use a clear vegetable glycerin, goat's milk, olive oil, or superfatted soap on the body only, unless you have normal to dry skin.

Selected Recipes for Mature Skin

My favorite toners for mature skin are a classic rosewater and glycerin blend and a lavender, chamomile, rose geranium, neroli, or rose tea or hydrosol mist. Try using a soothing and hydrating tea made with fennel seed, marshmallow root, or comfrey root as a body splash on occasion, especially when your skin is very dry.

Depending on the degree of dryness and the season, use an easily absorbed nutrient-rich lotion or cream for moisturizing both your face and body. An herbal elixir or facial oil containing carrot seed essential oil and rose hip seed base oil — key ingredients in Repair and Restore Remedy (page 168) and

valued for their highly regenerative and vitalizing properties — can be used as your only facial conditioning lubricant or as a first layer followed by lotion or cream if your skin is extra-thirsty. Avoid rose hip seed oil if your skin is oily; it can lead to breakouts.

SPECIAL INTENSIVE THERAPIES

To minimize the appearance of fine lines and wrinkles, fade age spots, and help maintain a smooth, refined appearance, twice weekly use a fruit-acid facial mask made from papaya, raspberry, strawberry, or pineapple purée (unless you have sensitive skin). A honey mask or moisturizing facial mask

Tips
ON MY SOAPBOX

Most soaps on the market today are highly alkaline and chock-full of synthetic chemicals, artificial fragrances, and antibacterial agents. They can strip your skin of its protective oils, leaving it dry, tight, flaky, itchy, and prone to dermatitis. Consequently, I generally recommend not using soap on your face and neck unless you have extremely oily skin; even then, you should only use soap in the warmest months.

I'm well aware that there are a number of people who swear by soap. You've used it all your life, you may say — every day, from head to toe, and even to wash your hair. That squeaky-clean feeling can make you feel ultra fresh! And because I know that old habits are hard to break, I won't insist that you give up your favorite bubbly bar. I do suggest, however, that you use the gentlest of soaps, such as those tolerated by sensitive skin: a superfatted, low-lathering bar; a goat's milk– or olive oil–based bar; a clear vegetable glycerin bar or liquid soap; or a nonirritating liquid castile soap designed for infants.

Regardless of your skin type, the most effective and nurturing way to cleanse your skin is to use a natural gel, lotion, or creamy cleanser; a finely ground oat, nut, or seed cleanser; or a clay-blend cleanser. If you wear heavy foundation makeup or work in a greasy environment, you can follow this with a second cleansing using a vegetable glycerin soap made specifically for the face.

deeply hydrates mature skin tissue and can be used daily. Enjoy a fennel seed, lavender, or calendula facial steam once a week to hydrate, cleanse impurities from the pores, and increase circulation.

Use a rich body oil following each shower or bath to seal in moisture and keep your skin supple, and apply eye cream as part of your daily skin care ritual. Because skin naturally thins and produces less oil as you age, by the time you reach your 50s, the already paper-thin skin surrounding your eyes has become even more translucent, drier, and wrinkle-prone. For youthful-looking eyes, don't squint but do invest in a snazzy pair of quality sunglasses!

Environmentally Damaged Skin

This skin type features premature lines, wrinkles, hyperpigmentation (freckles and age spots), ruddiness, rough texture, and uneven skin coloration, and it may begin to rear its ugly head somewhere around age 35. Much to the shock of those who have it, environmentally damaged skin often takes on the characteristics of mature skin. This skin type is reflective of the individual's lifestyle. People who tend to have environmentally damaged skin include smokers, heavy coffee and soda drinkers, people who consume large amounts of alcohol, routine recreational drug users, ocean-sport enthusiasts, sun worshippers, mountain climbers, tennis players, long-distance walkers or runners, or anybody who spends a lot of time in extreme outdoor climates. These people generally have skin that has been repeatedly severely dehydrated and

Selected Recipes for Environmentally Damaged Skin

weather beaten, and it may be impossible to return their skin to its former healthy, radiant suppleness because the collagen and elastin have lost their elasticity and flexibility.

Naturally fair, thin, dry skin is prone to environmental damage and can become painful, papery, parched skin that bleeds and tears easily as you age. If you have this skin type, be sure to take extra precautions when exposing yourself to the elements and do your best to make positive lifestyle choices that support skin health.

Environmentally damaged skin might have been oily or normal in its youth, but it's almost always at least normal to dry if not very dry after the age of 40.

CARE RECOMMENDATIONS

Because this type of skin is frequently sensitive and dry, read the sections on sensitive skin (page 29) and dry skin (page 25).

Each season brings its own challenges for environmentally damaged skin. Always remember that your skin needs deep hydration and constant sun protection. For the face and body, a nonirritating, mild, water-based lotion-type or creamy cleanser fortified with skin-nourishing oils such as jojoba, hazelnut, extra-virgin olive, sesame, sunflower, or macadamia nut deep-cleans and feeds your skin. Finely ground oat, nut, and seed cleansers and clay-blend cleansers are gentle skin foods that encourage softness and soothe irritation. If the skin on your body is dry, please avoid soap.

For toning, *mild* and *nondrying* are key words. A lavender, lemon balm, chamomile, or neroli hydrosol refreshes and removes any excess cleanser from the face. Never leave home without a spritzer bottle of purified water or your favorite hydrosol to quench your skin's thirst. Throughout the day, and every hour if desired, spray a light mist on your face. This keeps your makeup fresh and your skin from becoming flaky, dull, uncomfortable, and drab-looking.

For moisturizing, a lotion or cream enhanced with rose hip seed, coconut, sesame, macadamia nut, extra-virgin olive, sunflower, or jojoba oil helps feed, rejuvenate, tone, and support cell membrane functions within the skin of both the face and the body. An herbal facial elixir or facial oil with carrot seed, lavender, rosemary (ct. verbenon), neroli, or helichrysum essential oil helps stimulate new cell generation and encourages a brighter appearance.

SPECIAL INTENSIVE THERAPIES

See recommendations for dry skin (page 25).

Tips
CHEMICAL EXPOSURE AND YOUR SKIN

I wouldn't be doing my job as a holistic esthetician if I didn't at least mention the potential health risk of exposing your skin to synthetic chemicals. If your work environment or hobby requires you to breathe or handle petroleum-based products, welding gases, metal polishes, industrial or residential paints, solvents, toxic fumes, construction adhesives, coal or concrete dust, synthetic fertilizers, herbicides, pesticides, or any other "poison," please wear an appropriate mask and protective clothing — including gloves — at all times.

These chemicals and other "everyday" substances such as toxic household cleanser ingredients can leach into your bloodstream via your skin, resulting in heavy metal or toxic chemical poisoning. The side effects are not pleasant, and unless you undertake a blood test, the symptoms you may experience (such as headaches, nausea, weight gain, joint inflammation, dizziness, heart palpitations, nervousness, shortness of breath, high blood pressure, acne, eczema, mysterious rashes, and so on) will probably be diagnosed as another type of illness.

So protect yourself during exposure and be sure to cleanse your entire body regularly (and definitely before you go to sleep).

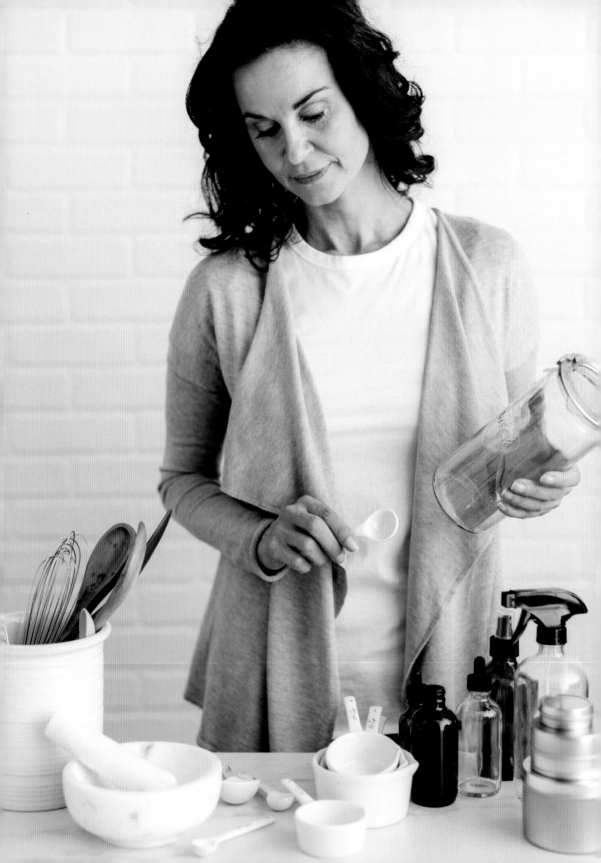

Chapter 2

CHOOSING YOUR TOOLS AND CONTAINERS

Making your own personal care products from natural ingredients is easy and soul-satisfying and can be a lot of fun. Only basic kitchen equipment and cooking skills are necessary for producing wonderfully fresh, body-nurturing creations. If you can boil water and make homemade salad dressing, mayonnaise, oatmeal, or pudding, then putting together these recipes will be as easy as pie.

This chapter includes three lists. The first identifies the equipment you will need for preparing your personal care recipes; the second covers storage container options based on which work best with a particular product; and the third includes applicators and cleansing tools, identifying some common and not-so-common items that will ensure you get the most from your creations.

"Cleanliness is next to godliness," as the saying goes, and whether you're preparing dinner for 12 or making personal care products, the same stringent sanitary precautions apply. Ideally, all implements necessary for formulation — pots, pans, spatulas, spoons, whisks, blender, knives, cutting board, storage containers, and every other tool — should be boiled or sterilized, but that's not practical or always possible. The next best alternative is to run through the dishwasher everything you'll be using or to soak implements for 15 minutes in very, very hot soapy water to which you've added 1 tablespoon of bleach for each gallon of water. Give your mixing implements and containers a good scrub and then allow them to air-dry thoroughly. The goal: to minimize the potential for harmful bacterial growth in your preservative-free products.

Your containers need to be as clean as possible, dry, and dust-free prior to pouring your newly made recipes into them.

I cannot emphasize enough that your containers need to be as clean as possible, dry, and dust-free prior to pouring your newly made recipes into them, and that your hands should be just-washed and dried as well. Introducing the tiniest bit of microbial contamination into your product can lead to the proliferation of mold or bacteria, and within a few weeks (depending on the warmth of your storage area), your lovely aromatic skin-pampering concoction will sport greenish-gray fuzz and you'll have to pitch it. What a waste! As with any worthwhile project you pursue in life, proper preparation is key.

PREPARATION TOOLS

Common kitchen tools are all you need to make the recipes in this book. Inexpensive tools will likely wear out quickly and have to be replaced; generally, middle-of-the-road quality is fine (unless you want to indulge yourself and purchase a top-of-the-line blender or coffee grinder for your projects). Here's a list of what you'll need.

Blender. This is great for whipping together creams and lotions in quantities of 2 cups or more. (When mixing smaller quantities, I find it difficult to get all the cream or lotion out of the bottom of the blender.) A blender can also be used to grind oatmeal, almonds, and sunflower seeds into meal, but a food processor or nut or seed grinder usually works better for this.

Bowls. You'll need a variety of sizes in glass, enamel, plastic, stainless steel, or ceramic. I use small bowls for mixing masks and single-serving facial scrubs and larger bowls for mixing the ingredients for herbal facial steams and body powders or making anything in quantity for myself or gift giving. Occasionally I use lidded plastic bowls for dry storage. Don't use plastic containers if you've

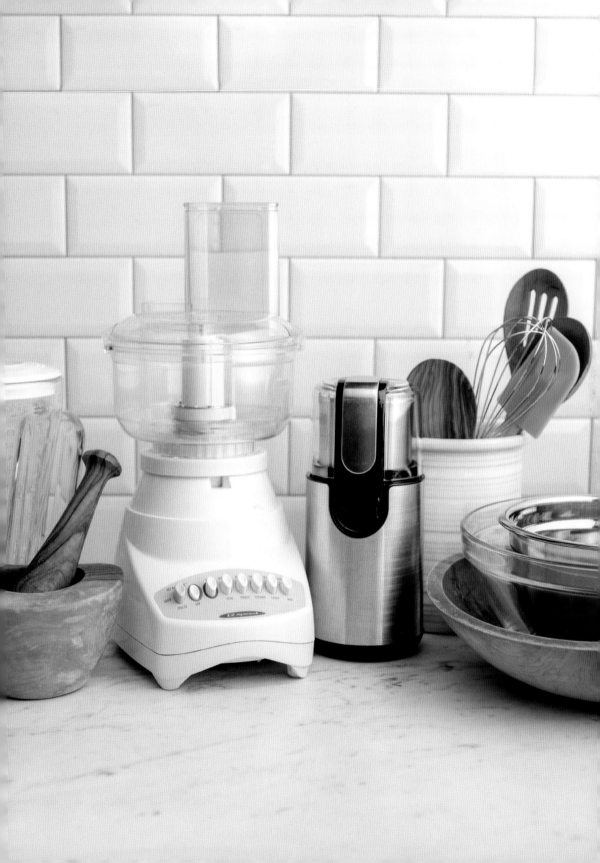

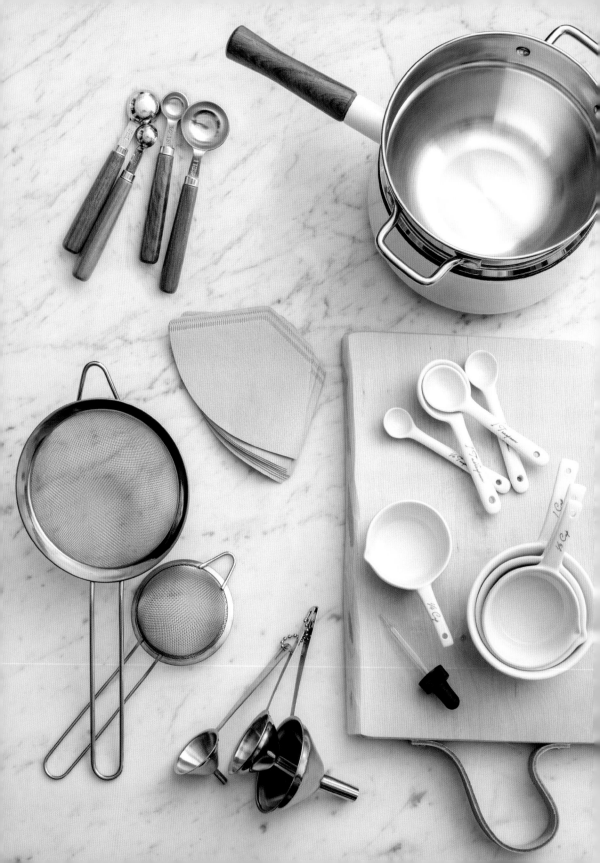

previously used them to store tomato sauce or anything strongly flavored or scented; plastic tends to absorb odors and flavors and can leach these into your products.

Coffee filters. An unbleached paper coffee filter is my filter of choice because it retains *all* herbal particulate matter when I am straining facial teas, astringents, toners, and herb-infused oils. Simply line a mesh strainer with a coffee filter and pour in your liquid. Perfectly clean herbal infusions will strain through. A doubled layer of cheesecloth, the toe of an old nylon stocking, a muslin bag or piece of muslin fabric, or any finely woven mesh bag makes a good substitute, though some herbal particulate matter may filter through, and then the product will require a second round of straining.

Coffee grinder. This kitchen gadget gets more use than any other piece of equipment I own aside from my blender. I use it to grind oats, nuts, sunflower seeds, and dried flowers and lightweight leafy herbs to the precise texture I want. Be sure to use separate grinders for your personal care products and your coffee! Coffee beans leave a lingering flavor and aroma in the grinder that will permeate your natural cosmetic ingredients, thereby tainting your creations.

Cutting board. You'll need a cutting board for slicing and dicing miscellaneous items. Always keep a separate board for use with any dairy, meat, poultry, or fish products. Remember to keep your boards

scrupulously clean at all times; they can harbor bacteria in grooved and nicked areas.

Double boiler. A double boiler is a two-part pot designed to moderate the heat that comes off a stovetop burner. The bottom section holds simmering water, while the ingredients go into the top part. If you don't have a "proper" double boiler, you can achieve the same results by setting a heat-resistant glass or metal bowl over a saucepan containing simmering water. I occasionally use a double boiler to melt hard or thick ingredients, such as wax, cocoa butter, shea butter, or coconut oil, and to warm liquid oils when making various creams, lotions, and lip balms. The advantage of a double boiler is that it produces a gentle, even, relatively low heat, making it impossible to scorch or boil your ingredients if you happen to get called away from the kitchen or get distracted. Usually, though, I simply heat my ingredients in a regular stainless steel pan over low heat, stirring occasionally. I always use a timer and keep an eye on what I'm doing!

   Note: When making products that contain fatty ingredients such as oils, waxes, or butters, low heat is the key. If you simmer, overheat, boil, or scorch these ingredients, they'll be ruined. In this case, the saying "a watched pot never boils" is a good thing! In making body care products, always keep a watchful eye on what you're doing.

Dropper (glass). Sometimes called an eye-dropper, a dropper is a tool used for measuring liquids (like essential oils) by the drop. Glass is preferable because, unlike plastic, it doesn't retain scent or color, and some essential oils, especially citrus oils, will rapidly degrade plastic and rubber. After each use, rinse the dropper with hot water, then pour isopropyl rubbing alcohol or 95 percent ethyl alcohol (inexpensive 80-proof vodka works great, though, if that's all you have on hand) through it to sterilize it. Allow the dropper to dry completely before using it again.

Most essential oils come in 10- or 15-milliliter bottles, with "drop-by-drop" orifice-reducer inserts for easy dispensing, eliminating the need for an additional dropper, but larger bottles are often sealed with a simple screw top, and you'll need a dropper for dispensing their contents.

Food processor (full-size or small model). This can be used for mixing larger amounts (usually 2 cups or more) of facial and body scrubs, facial masks, and body powders, or for making finely ground oatmeal, almond meal, and sunflower seed meal.

Funnel. This comes in handy when you're pouring liquid recipes into narrow-necked storage bottles. If you don't have an actual funnel, you can make one in a snap from aluminum foil, and because herbal liquids pass through a funnel so quickly, there is no real risk of aluminum leaching into your product, as there is with using aluminum pots and pans.

Measuring cups and spoons. Preparing creams and lotions requires exact measurements, which is where these come in handy. Glass, plastic, or stainless steel is fine. Some herbalists I know use incrementally marked glass measuring cups (or bowls) in the microwave (versus pots on a stovetop) to warm and melt all their ingredients. Glass measuring cups or bowls of this kind are easy to hold (most have a handle), and because of the easy-to-read measurement markings, you can be sure you've measured ingredients accurately. Product perfection is virtually guaranteed — as long as you don't overheat the ingredients!

Mortar and pestle (with a mortar approximately 6 inches in diameter). I use this tool to crush fennel seeds, to crush fresh herbs and flowers to extract their juices, and to mash ripe papaya, banana, pineapple chunks, and ripe berries. A mortar and pestle is also handy for combining essential oils and unscented powder mixtures for herbal body powders.

Pans. I use myriad sizes that vary from tiny 1-cup pans to 6-quart ones, in enamel, glass, or stainless steel. *Please do not use pans made from aluminum or copper.* These metals can react with the herbs, fruits, resins, and acidic liquids in your recipes and leach the aluminum and copper into the products you're making. Aluminum, in particular, is not good for your skin. It can also affect the beneficial qualities of the herbs and can discolor the end product.

Paring knives. Always keep several very sharp blades at your disposal for cutting and peeling just about anything.

Rubber spatulas. These are perfect for scooping out creams, lotions, balms, salves, and butters from any type of container. I find that long-handled, narrow spatulas come in handy when I need to occasionally free up the oil- and wax-clogged blender blades or scrape down the sides of the blender container as I mix thick creams and lotions.

Spoons and stirring utensils. One small and one medium wooden spoon are indispensable. A stainless steel iced-tea spoon works well for blending liquids in tiny pans or beating small amounts of face cream. Wooden chopsticks, 1/2-inch-diameter dowels, and the handles of wooden spoons are useful for poking into tall containers, as well as for dredging sludgy oil- or alcohol-sodden herbs from the bottom of saucepans or canning jars.

Strainer. You'll need a bamboo, wire, or fabric mesh strainer for straining herbs from liquids in various recipes.

Whisks. I use a small, slender whisk for whipping and blending creams and lotions in a saucepan. It works best for blending small amounts, while a blender or food processor works better for larger recipes. I use a large whisk for gently stirring body powder blends or larger quantities of body and facial scrubs.

STORAGE CONTAINERS

The more attractive and user-friendly the containers you use for storing your handmade personal care products, the better. Aesthetic appeal is important — especially if you intend to give your products as gifts. See Resources (page 237) for mail-order companies and Internet sources that sell storage containers. For these special products, a recycled mustard jar will not do! Here are some storage container ideas.

Bottles (1/2 ounce to 16 ounces). I use dark glass and plastic. These are great for storing anything liquid, including base oils, astringents and toners, body oils, and facial elixirs. I always use glass, though, when creating and storing larger amounts of vodka- and witch hazel–based herbal extracts. If you're using glass, choose amber, dark green, or cobalt blue, especially if the product will be exposed to bright light for an extended period of time. Dark glass helps preserve the volatile natural properties of herbs, base oils, and essential oils. When you're traveling, or if your home is full of small children and pets, plastic bottles might be preferable. If they are clear, be sure to store them away from light once they are filled.

Note: If a recipe specifically indicates the use of a glass container for storage, please heed that instruction.

Canning jars (1/2 pint to 1 gallon). These are suitable for storing dried herbs (store them out of direct light) and for making solar-infused oils. The half-pint size is perfect for packaging scrubs, masks, and dry herbal cleansers to give to friends. Slap on your custom label and voilà! You've got a beautiful present.

Cream jars (¼ ounce to 8 ounces). These are perfect for storing creams, lotions, balms, body butters, salves, and facial and body scrubs. These jars are available in glass or plastic.

Plastic tubs. Plastic food storage containers with airtight lids can be used to store dried herbs, powder blends, and dry cleansers, scrubs, and masks.

Shaker jars. Shaker jars are great for storing herbal body and foot powders. You can use the small plastic and glass shaker jars that hold culinary herbs and spices; just wash them thoroughly after you've used up the seasoning! I sometimes store dry facial and body scrub mixtures in these containers as well.

Spritzer bottles. These are good for packaging astringents, toners, or any recipe that requires a spray application. You can find them in glass or plastic.

Squeeze bottles. These plastic bottles make great storage containers for astringents, toners, and body oils.

Tins (¼ ounce to 8 ounces or larger). Tins have a lovely old-fashioned appeal and look very attractive when decorated with a custom-made label, making them great gift-giving containers. I like to use these to store dried herbs, body powders with a silky-soft applicator puff, and dry facial and body scrubs. They're relatively airtight and keep out both bugs and light.

Ziplock freezer bags. Dried herbs are best stored in tightly sealed jars, tins, or plastic tubs, but ziplock freezer bags are a reasonable and inexpensive alternative, and they're fine for baking soda, powdered clays, ground meals (such as sunflower, almond, and oat), Epsom salt, beeswax pastilles, cocoa butter wafers, and other dry ingredients. If you do use them to store herbs, keep them in a very dry, dark, cool place and use the herbs within a year. If you use ziplock bags to store ground meals, keep them in the freezer and use within one year, as the inherent fats quickly turn rancid.

Note: The slide-lock freezer bags are *not* airtight; use the double-zipper style instead.

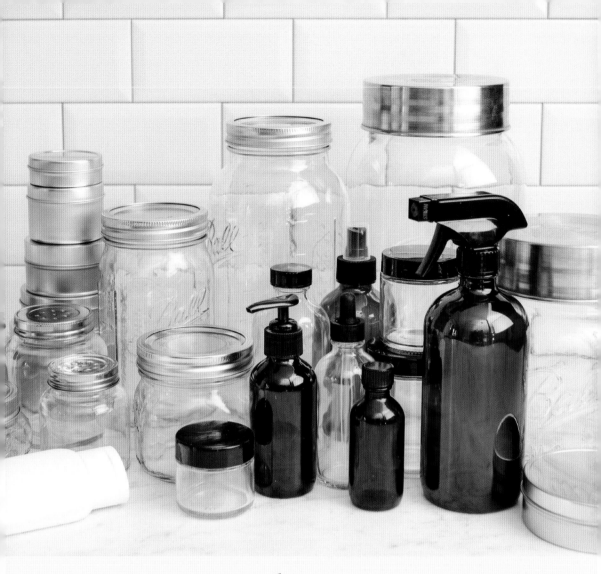

Tips
RECYCLING STORAGE CONTAINERS

If you plan to recycle previously used glass or plastic containers for storage purposes, be sure to wash them thoroughly first. You can either run them through the dishwasher or allow them to soak for 15 minutes in very hot, soapy water with a splash of bleach added. After they've soaked, scrub thoroughly, rinse, and allow them to air-dry completely. Do not store your cosmetics in containers that have previously held medicine, poisons, household cleansers (other than dishwashing liquid), spoiled foods, or fertilizers. Use your own good judgment about which containers are safe to use, and never reuse a lid that is rusty or was previously covered with mold.

GLASS VERSUS PLASTIC

Generally speaking, dark glass (amber, cobalt blue, or dark green) is the best option when it comes to storing your personal care products and home remedies, as the tint helps preserve the volatile properties contained within the botanical liquids against the damaging effects of bright light. Plus, glass won't react with the chemical constituents in the botanicals. Essential oils should *always* be stored in glass, and if you are decanting pure, undiluted essential oils from larger to small containers, dark glass is a must.

I prefer glass and love its heft, look, and feel. However, in some cases, it's impossible, impractical, or downright inconvenient to use glass for your natural concoctions, such as when you are traveling, if you have small children and pets, or if you are storing containers in the shower or carrying them in a purse, briefcase, or backpack. Plastic can be a viable option, but you have to use the right type, and essential oils *must always be diluted* before being stored in plastic containers because they can degrade the plastic over time, leaching harmful chemicals into the product. If you decide to use plastic containers, here's what to look for:

 PET plastic: Polyethylene terephthalate is safe, nontoxic, strong, lightweight, flexible, and recyclable. It is available in standard clear or clear cobalt blue, green, or amber bottles and jars, plus some solid colors. A #1 recycle symbol on a plastic container indicates that it is made of PET. When I must use a plastic container, PET plastic is my favorite.

 HDPE plastic: High-density polyethylene is safe, nontoxic, superstrong, lightweight, flexible, recyclable, impact-resistant, weather-resistant, and long-lasting. It is available in bottles and jars, typically opaque, but also in a few solid colors. The #2 recycle symbol on a container indicates that it is made of HDPE.

APPLICATION AND CLEANSING TOOLS

The following handy-to-have items make application and removal of many personal care products more effective and enjoyable. These items are not required, but all are useful.

Complexion brush. This brush, either manual or with a motorized rotating head or oscillating bristles, is usually about the size of your palm or may have a short handle with the bristles forming a 1- to 1¹/₂-inch-diameter circular pattern. The synthetic bristles should be very, very soft, akin to an infant's hairbrush or slightly firmer. Use a complexion brush much as you would a washcloth to gently exfoliate the skin on your face and neck — but steer clear of the eye area — while simultaneously cleansing with your foaming or creamy cleanser. Store your brush in such a way that it will dry thoroughly between uses. A consistently damp brush will encourage mold growth and will destroy the area where the bristles attach to the base. Be sure to give the brush a thorough washing with soap and water at least once per week.

Cosmetic fan brush. This is a slender-handled cosmetic brush approximately 6 to 8 inches long, with fan-shaped synthetic or natural bristles. Estheticians frequently use these brushes to "paint" masks onto the face for even distribution or to apply thinned yogurt or fruit pulp.

Cotton balls or cotton squares/rounds. There are so many uses for these that I can't mention them all here. I like to soak them in cold milk or herb tea and apply them as soothing eye pads or soak them with oil and use them to remove stubborn eye makeup. Many people use them to apply astringent or toner or moisten them with cleanser to gently cleanse the face and neck. I prefer to buy 100 percent cotton (preferably organic) balls or squares or cut my own from rolled cotton, which is sometimes called beautician's cotton.

Facial chamois cloth. This is a synthetic version of a washcloth — about the same size, rather thin, slightly rubbery, and very soft. I highly recommend it for cleansing ultrasensitive acneic or environmentally damaged skin. It makes a perfect cloth for the delicate skin of an infant or very thin, papery, fragile, elderly skin.

Loofah. A loofah is actually the dried skeleton of a gourd. It's wonderful to use with foaming body cleansers and is excellent for daily exfoliation of dry skin buildup on the body but is too rough for use on the face. Loofahs tend to retain moisture and can mold easily, so after use, be sure to place yours in an upright position where it can dry and receive plenty of air circulation.

Sea sponge. Small sea sponges are great for face cleansing, and the larger ones are handy in the bath or shower when applying foaming

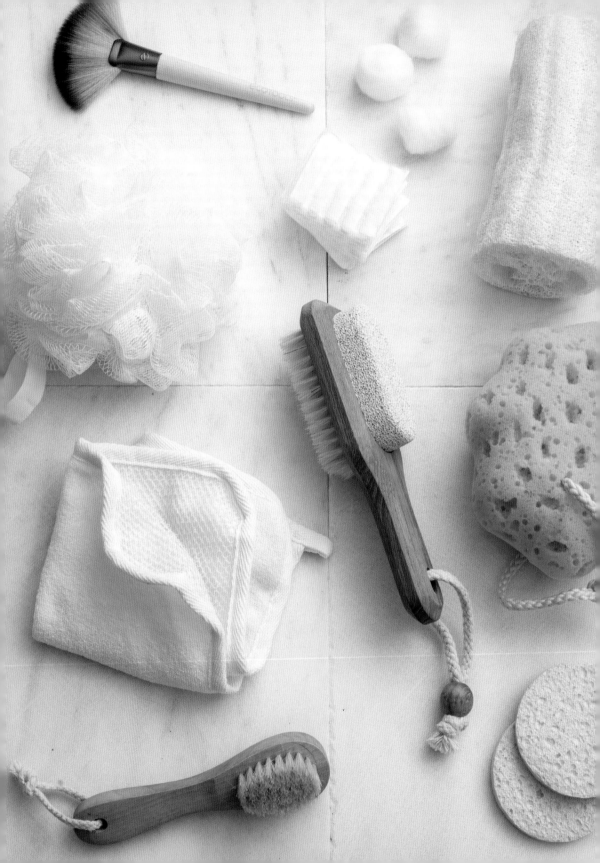

cleansers. (**Note:** A little foaming cleanser goes a long way when applied with a sponge versus a washcloth.) Like loofahs, sea sponges can mold easily. Please find a storage place where yours can dry between uses.

Tissues. Some people use tissues for everything under the sun, including to blot excess perspiration and oil from the face, to blot or remove lipstick, and to remove cleansing creams and lotions and eye makeup when a washcloth is unavailable. If you're in need of either invigoration or relaxation, place a drop or two of the appropriate essential oil onto a tissue and inhale, or tuck the tissue into your shirt or under your pillow at night. Use only unscented white tissues — dyes and fragrances may irritate delicate skin. For cosmetic purposes, avoid ultrasoft, puffy, lotion-impregnated tissues, which can be very fibrous and can leave tiny bits of annoying fuzz on your face and lips.

Washing puff or cleansing pad. This soft pad is usually a circular piece of 3- or 5-inch foam covered with fine-textured terry cloth. It works just like a washcloth but tends to be less fibrous and is thus gentler on the skin.

Tips

2 TABLESPOONS = 1 OUNCE

Math and Kitchen Cosmetology

Don't panic and bite your nails because the word *math* appears here! Whether you're a beginner or an experienced cosmetic cook, it's good to know a few simple measurement equivalents. Commit these to memory and they'll make preparation of your products a bit quicker, especially if you want to customize a recipe or make a larger or smaller batch than what a recipe is designed to make.

BY THE TABLESPOON

⅓ tablespoon	= 1 teaspoon	
1 tablespoon	= 3 teaspoons	= ½ fluid ounce
4 tablespoons	= ¼ cup	= 2 fluid ounces
16 tablespoons	= 1 cup	= 8 fluid ounces

BY THE OUNCE

1 fluid ounce	= 2 tablespoons	
8 fluid ounces	= 1 cup	
16 fluid ounces	= 2 cups	= 1 pint
32 fluid ounces	= 4 cups	= 2 pints or 1 quart
1 gallon	= 16 cups	= 4 quarts

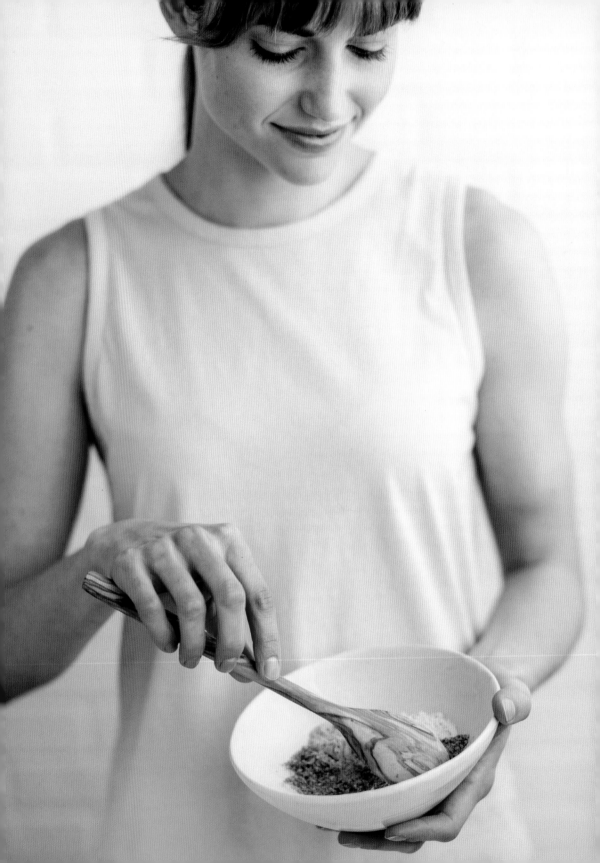

Chapter 3

BASIC
TECHNIQUES

All of the recipes in the following chapters can be made in your home kitchen. Many require only a couple ingredients to be stirred together, which can be done in less than 5 minutes. Others call for steeping some dried or fresh herbs in a liquid mixture for 2 weeks. A few involve heating ingredients and then blending them together, and some involve grinding nuts and seeds. But none of my recipes are complicated. If you know how to make tea, salad dressing, or mayonnaise, you know how to make natural skin care products!

The pages that follow provide an overview of the techniques you'll use to make some of the recipes in part two (page 63). These particular techniques have a bit of a learning curve, which is why they are highlighted here. Look through these methods before you start trying the recipes, but also remember to read each recipe carefully to ensure you understand the steps involved. With a little attention to detail and some practice, you soon will be creating cleansers, astringents, toners, scrubs, facial elixirs, balms, body creams, and more that rival high-end commercial products.

Making Skin Care Tinctures

About half of the astringent and toner recipes in this book require tincturing — or using alcohol and/or witch hazel as the extractive substance — to draw out the remedial properties from the herbs with which they are combined. The process typically takes 2 weeks to complete, during which time the mixing jar must be stored in a cool, dark cabinet to steep. This is a very simple yet effective method of making gentle herbal tinctures for skin care.

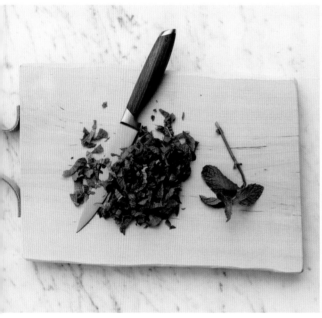
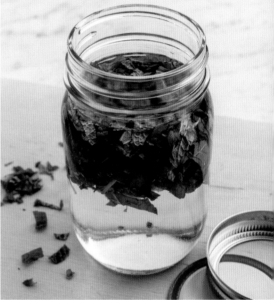

1. If you are using herbs, prepare them according to the recipe's instructions.

2. Combine all the ingredients in a glass jar and seal tightly. Shake well.

3. Steep for the specified length of time.

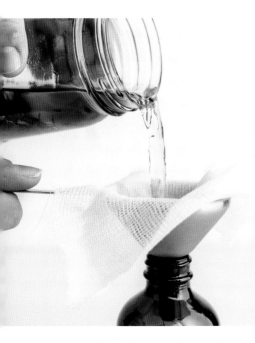

4. Strain out the herbs according to the recipe's instructions.

5. Pour tincture into storage container(s), cap, label, and date.

SAFETY FIRST

Many of the recipes in this book will look and smell edible because the majority of ingredients used are edible, but this does not mean that any particular product here is safe to consume, especially if it contains essential oils, vodka- or witch hazel–infused herbal extracts, or powdered clay. If a facial recipe happens to drip into your mouth, that is generally okay, though. Please, for safety's sake, clearly label and date all your personal care products and keep them out of the reach of children and pets.

While making your personal care products, if any of the solutions or mixtures come into contact with your eyes, promptly flood them with an unscented, bland fatty oil such as almond, sunflower, jojoba, olive, corn, soybean, peanut, or generic vegetable oil (especially in the case of essential oil accidents), or water or cold milk, repeatedly. If any irritation continues, see your health care provider as soon as possible.

Preparing and Using Facial Steams

For some of my skin care products, the preparation of the recipe takes much more time than the application. The opposite is true for facial steams. Making a facial steam is almost as easy as boiling water. Follow the instructions below for using your facial steam to reap the full benefits.

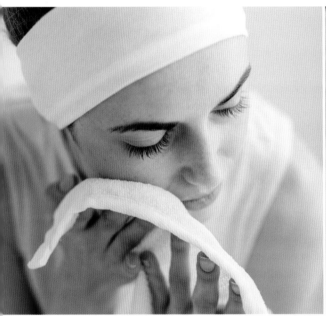

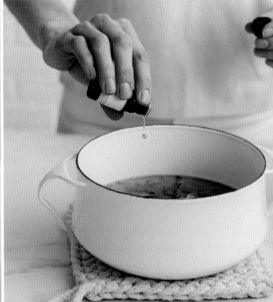

1. To prepare for a facial steam, first thoroughly cleanse your skin.

2. Bring 3 cups of distilled or purified water to a boil. If a recipe calls for vinegar, boil it with the water. Remove the liquid from the heat, add the herbs, cover, and let it steep for 5 minutes. Then stir in any other ingredients called for in the recipe, such as base oil or essential oil.

Achieving Beautiful Skin, Naturally

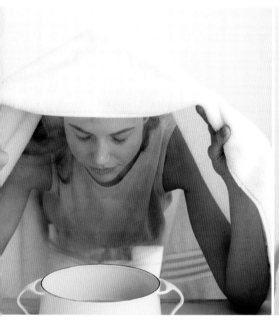
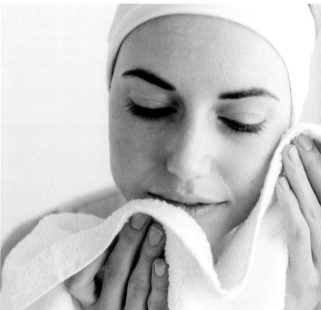

3. Place the pot of infused, steaming herbs on a heat-safe, stable surface where you can lean over it comfortably for 10 minutes, such as a table or countertop. Remove the cover from the pan and drape a large bath towel over your head and shoulders and the steaming herb pot to create a tent.

4. With your eyes closed and your face 10 to 12 inches from the pot (to avoid burn-ing your skin), breathe deeply and relax. Keep your eyes closed during the entire steam. If you feel overheated, you can lift a corner of the towel, as shown above, to vent steam as needed.

5. When you're finished, splash your face and neck with tepid water, followed by a few splashes of cool water. Pat your skin until it is almost dry. For a full facial treatment, finish by using a mask and moisturizer.

Making Balms

The key to making smooth-textured body balms is melting the fats slowly, with low heat. While the steps below show you the basic process, be sure to read each recipe carefully, as mixing and cooling times vary.

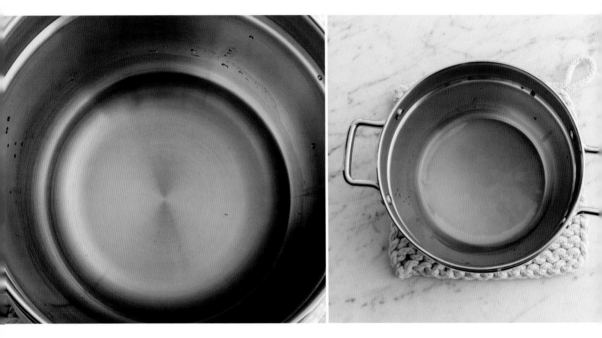

1. In a small saucepan over low heat or in a double boiler, warm all of the base oils, waxes, and butters *except* vitamin E oil and essential oil, until the solids are just melted.

2. Remove from the heat and gently stir with a small spoon according to the recipe's instructions, then allow the mixture to cool for the amount of time specified in each recipe.

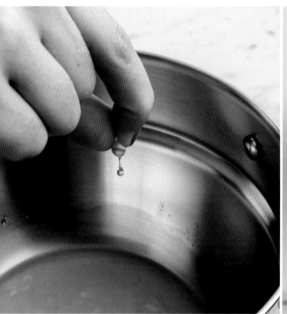

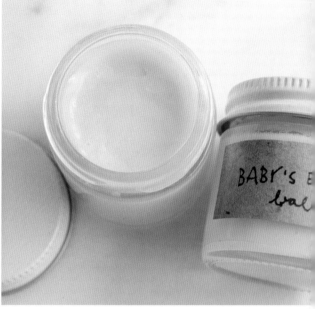

3. Add the vitamin E oil capsule(s) (pierce the capsule skin and squeeze the contents into the mix) and essential oil, and stir to blend.

4. Pour into storage container(s) and cap, label, and date. Allow the mixture to set for 12 hours or overnight.

Tips
COOKING

When heating and melting various oils, waxes, butters, and water-based ingredients for blending, please use the *low* setting on your stove and place the ingredients in a small saucepan, or use a double boiler or the microwave. (If you choose to use the microwave, warm ingredients for only 10 to 15 seconds at a time to avoid overheating.)

   Never allow the herbal liquid or oil/butter/wax mixture to get too hot or bubble or simmer, no matter what "cooking" method you choose. Gently warm them just enough for the solids to melt and the vegetable glycerin (when called for) to dissolve in the water or herbal liquid.

Making Creams
and Lotions

Creating luscious cleansing creams, body lotions, and body butters is the most involved process in this book, but don't be intimidated by the number of steps below! You'll gently heat up some fats and base oils, just like you might melt butter, then add these to your blender to cool for a short time. Next, you'll slowly drizzle in a blend of water-based ingredients to form an emulsion. The process is similar to making mayonnaise or aioli — and the results are just as rich!

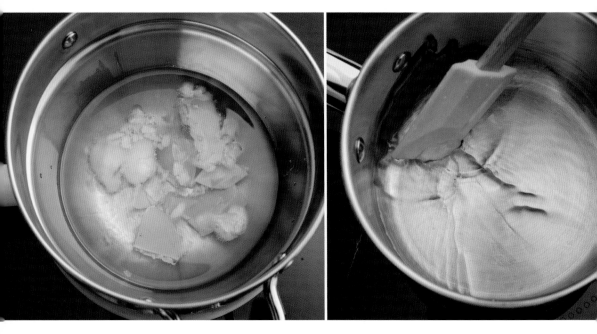

1. In a small saucepan over low heat or in a double boiler, warm the fatty ingredients — including base oils, butters, and beeswax, but excluding vitamin E oil — until the solids are just melted.

2. In another small pan, gently warm the watery ingredients — which, depending on the recipe, may include water, aloe vera juice, tea, hydrosol, and vegetable glycerin — and stir a few times until the glycerin dissolves in the liquid.

Achieving Beautiful Skin, Naturally

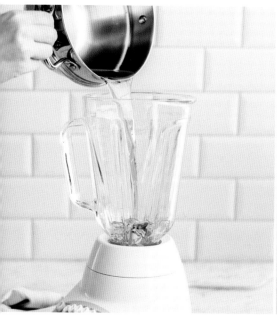
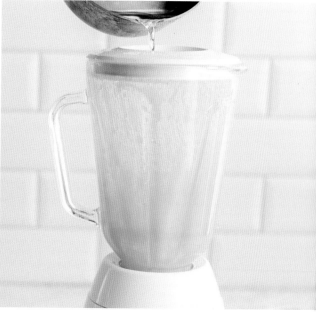

3. Remove both pans from the heat. Pour the oil/butter/wax mixture into a blender and allow it to cool for approximately 20 minutes, or until it begins to turn slightly opaque. The time will vary depending on the temperature of your kitchen.

Do not walk away and forget what you're doing and allow this mixture to get too thick, or else it will not blend properly and you may have a difficult time getting it out of your blender. Been there, done that!

4. Place the lid on the blender and remove the piece in the center to allow pouring. Turn the blender on medium speed. Slowly drizzle the mixture of watery ingredients through the center of the lid into the vortex of swirling fats below. Almost immediately the cream will turn off-white to very pale yellow and will begin to thicken.

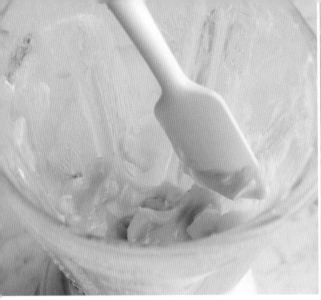
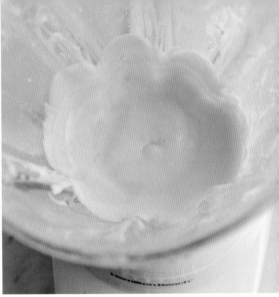

5. Blend for 10 to 15 seconds, or until all the watery mixture has been added, then turn off the blender and check the consistency of the cream. It should have a smooth, glossy texture.

6. If the watery mixture is not properly combining with the fatty mixture, give the cream a few stirs with a spatula, being sure to scrape down any cream residue from the sides of the blender container. Then replace the lid and blend on medium speed for another 5 to 10 seconds. Repeat this process once or twice more, if necessary, until the cream is smooth.

To Store

No refrigeration is required if you use up the cream within 60 to 90 days. It will keep best if stored in a dark, cool cabinet. If your storage area is very warm, please use up the cream within 4 weeks for maximum potency and freshness. On the day that you notice any mold growing in your container, toss it out and make a fresh batch.

If, after a few hours or days, water begins to separate from your cream, don't worry.

You can pour off the watery liquid and use the resulting super-thick product as a foot, elbow, or knee balm. The mixture can separate if the temperature of the fatty ingredients and that of the water ingredients are not relatively equal and cool enough when the two portions are blended.

Achieving Beautiful Skin, Naturally

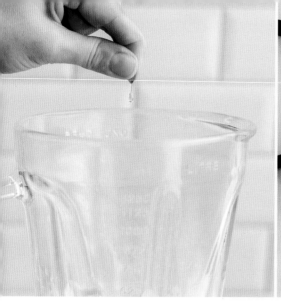
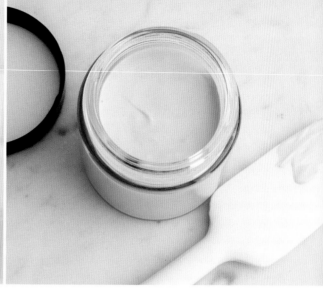

7. Turn off the blender and add the vitamin E oil capsule(s) by piercing the capsule skin and squeezing the contents into the cream and the essential oils. Put the lid back on, then blend for another 5 seconds or so, until the cream is smooth and thick.

Note: If the temperature of your kitchen is above 76°F (24°C), the cream will maintain a softer consistency. (Coconut oil turns from solid to liquid at 76°F.) If your kitchen is below 76°F, the cream will be firmer.

8. Pour the finished cream into storage container(s). Lightly cover each container with a paper towel and allow the cream to cool for about 30 minutes before capping and labeling.

Getting the Right Consistency

Blending cleansing creams, facial creams, body lotions, and body butters takes practice. You're attempting to combine oily and fatty ingredients with water-based ones — which naturally repel each other — and get them to stabilize chemically and form an emulsion. Just as occurs with homemade mayonnaise, hollandaise sauce, or gravy, though, when watery ingredients and fats are blended properly and at the right temperatures, magic happens! A fabulous cream appears right before your eyes.

In order for everything to blend properly, the fatty mixture should be approximately the same temperature as the watery mixture — about body temperature or slightly cooler.

To make a cream thicker or firmer, add a tad more beeswax, cocoa butter, or shea butter. Experiment and see which one produces the consistency and texture you like best. Shea butter will always remain softer than beeswax or cocoa butter.

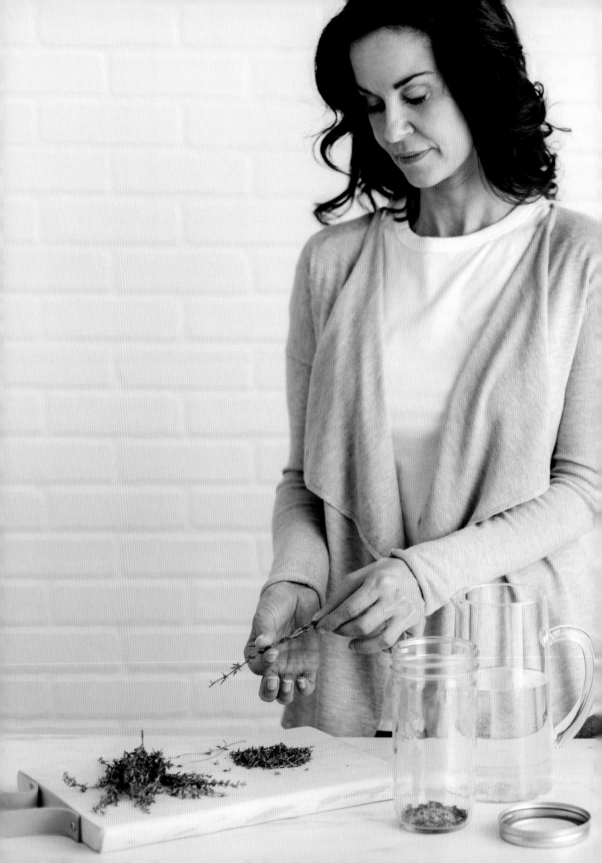

Part Two

MAKING YOUR SKIN CARE *Products*

Your skin needs consistent TLC in order to maintain its health, smooth texture, resiliency, suppleness, and comfort as you age. Here you'll learn how to take care of your skin naturally from the outside in. The recipes run the gamut from cleansers, astringents, masks, and scrubs to rich moisturizers, body oils, and balms, plus all-important natural sun protection. The end products are so delightfully soothing and pampering that you'll want to lavish as much attention on your body as possible. Remember: *pampering* is not a dirty word; it's a downright necessity!

Before we begin, it's important to note a few points about the recipes themselves:

Each ingredient is included in a recipe for a specific reason — it contributes to the integrity of the final product.

As your knowledge of personal care products grows and you gain blending experience, I encourage you to use the recipes here more as guidelines so that you can customize some to suit your personal specifications. As your skills develop, experiment and add your own special touch to each.

In the chapters that follow, you'll find my favorite tried-and-true formulas for natural personal care products for the face, eyes, body, feet, and hands. Be creative and enjoy the process!

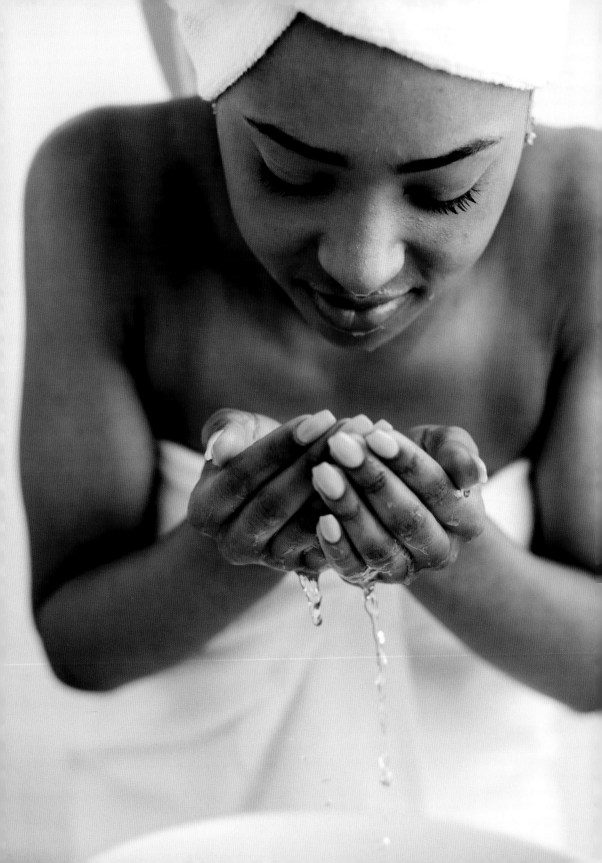

Chapter 4

CLEAN

Recipes for Cleansers, Astringents, and Toners

All of the recipes in this chapter help keep your face clean, hydrated, and healthy, gently and naturally. Each type of product has a specific purpose and benefit, and some are better for certain skin types than others. A few require just two or three ingredients and can be quickly produced, while others are more involved, necessitating the brewing of herbal extracts, creating natural liquid soap mixtures, heating base oils, butters, and waxes, and blending creams. Simply choose the recipes that suit your current skin type and particular needs, keeping in mind your environment and lifestyle habits.

Facial Cleansers

Facial cleansers are designed to remove everyday dirt and grime that collects on your skin's surface and in your facial pores. Creamy and oil-based cleansers are frequently used as an initial makeup cleanser because they do a better job of removing makeup than foaming, powdered, or clay-based products. Many people who wear foundation makeup or work in a greasy or dirty environment follow up with a second cleansing using the same product or a foaming cleanser, a mild soap (such as one made from fatty goat's milk), a clay-based cleanser, or a powdered soap-free cleanser. All of the recipes that follow are very gentle and nourishing and do a thorough job of cleansing.

Storage Tips

The cleansing creams here contain no preservatives except for natural vitamin E oil and essential oils, and thus they have a relatively short shelf life. They generally require no refrigeration if used up within 60 to 90 days, unless your storage area is very warm. If cleansing cream is stored unopened in the refrigerator and the product is untouched, it may keep for up to 6 months or more. Please note that though refrigeration may change the product's texture a bit, it will not affect its potency.

Foaming, oil-based, and powdered cleansers need no refrigeration and generally have a much longer shelf life than cleansing creams and lotions. Specific refrigeration and storage requirements are included with each recipe.

CLASSIC ROSEWATER *and* GLYCERIN FRESHENING CLEANSER

SKIN TYPES RECOMMENDED FOR
all

This product is best to use as a light, freshening cleanser on your makeup-free days, after you work out, or anytime you feel a bit sweaty. It does not remove makeup, but it does double as a moisturizing toner for parched skin: it's very gentle and soothing and leaves skin feeling soft and smelling like roses.

YIELD: 1 cup

PREP TIME: 10 minutes

- 1 cup rose hydrosol
- 2 teaspoons vegetable glycerin

TO MAKE

Combine the hydrosol and glycerin in your plastic or glass bottle or spritzer. Shake vigorously for about 30 seconds to blend. Label and date.

TO STORE

No refrigeration is required, but for maximum freshness and potency, please use within 6 to 12 months. Store in a dark, cool cabinet.

TO APPLY

Anytime your skin needs freshening, apply this liquid cleanser with a washcloth or cleansing pad. Use 1 to 2 teaspoons per application.

Use daily. Follow with moisturizer, if desired.

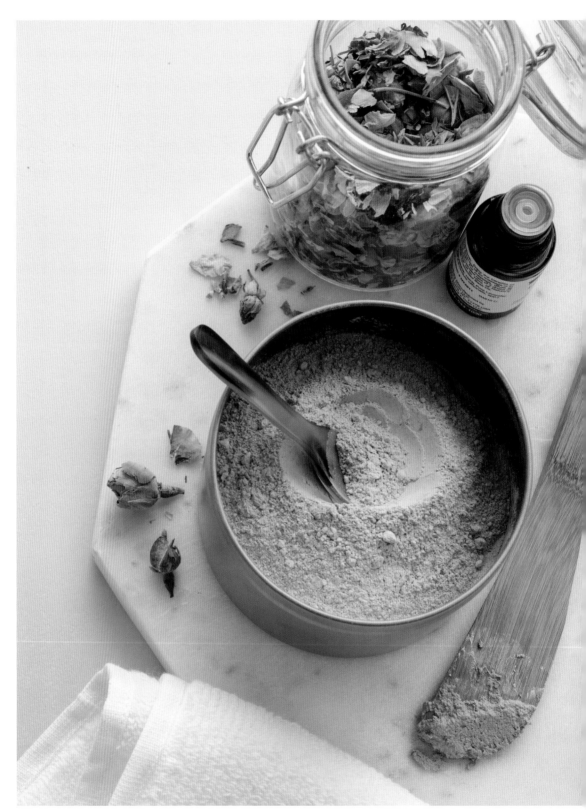

LAVENDER *and* ROSES GENTLE CLEANSING POWDER

SKIN TYPES RECOMMENDED FOR
all

This is a lightly fragranced cleanser for those who wear minimal makeup. It also doubles as a face mask and gentle exfoliant; simply spread it on cleansed skin, let it dry for 20 to 30 minutes, then rinse. If you prevent moisture from entering the container, this cleanser will not spoil.

YIELD: 1 cup

PREP TIME: 10 to 15 minutes

- ½ cup powdered white clay
- ⅓ cup plus 1 tablespoon finely ground oatmeal or oat flour
- 1 tablespoon powdered lavender buds
- 1 tablespoon powdered rose petals
- 10 drops lavender essential oil
- 5 drops rose otto or geranium essential oil

TO MAKE

Combine the clay, oatmeal, powdered lavender buds, and powdered rose petals in a medium bowl and stir to blend. Add the essential oils by the drop, and stir again to thoroughly incorporate. Scoop the mixture into a storage container, label, and date.

TO STORE

No refrigeration is required, but for maximum freshness and potency, please use within 6 months. Store in a cool, dry place.

TO APPLY

Scoop 2 teaspoons of powdered cleanser into a small bowl or the palm of your hand and add 2 teaspoons of water, coconut water, coconut milk, almond milk, or dairy milk. Stir until the mixture forms a spreadable paste, and allow this paste to thicken for a minute.

Using your fingers, apply the entire mixture over your face and throat (avoiding the eye area). Massage in circular motions for a minute. Rinse with warm water.

Use daily. Follow with astringent or toner.

REFRESHING SKIN WASH

This product doubles as an especially invigorating body wash for oily and normal skin and also makes an effective antibacterial hand soap. It's excellent for use on back acne, and you can dilute it by half with distilled or purified water and use it as a shampoo for oily hair.

YIELD: 2 cups

PREP TIME: 10 minutes

- 1 teaspoon hazelnut or jojoba oil
- 5 drops green myrtle essential oil
- 5 drops palmarosa essential oil
- 5 drops peppermint essential oil
- 5 drops tea tree essential oil
- 1 (16-ounce) bottle unscented liquid castile soap

Try substituting lavender, lemon, thyme (ct. linalool), or geranium essential oil for *any* of the essential oils listed above.

TO MAKE

Add the hazelnut oil and essential oils to the bottle of castile soap. Shake vigorously. Store the finished product right in the bottle. Label and date.

TO STORE

No refrigeration is required, but for maximum freshness and potency, please use within 1 year. Store in a dark, cool cabinet or in the shower.

TO APPLY

Shake well before each use. Moisten your face with warm water. Using a soft, damp cloth, a cleansing pad, or your fingers, apply approximately ½ to 1 teaspoon of the skin wash over your entire face and throat. Castile soap is highly concentrated, so a little goes a long way. Rinse with warm water.

Use daily. Follow with astringent or toner.

EVER-SO-GENTLE SOAP-LOVER'S FACE and BODY WASH

SKIN TYPES RECOMMENDED FOR all, except very dry or environmentally damaged

This recipe dilutes the castile soap by 50 percent with skin-pampering hydrosols, thus creating a very gentle liquid soap product for virtually all skin types. It makes an effective cleanser for the entire body, with a soothing, subtle floral scent. I like to use this formula when my normal-to-dry skin becomes seasonally oily in the summer.

YIELD: 2 cups

PREP TIME: 10 minutes

- 1 (8-ounce) bottle unscented liquid castile soap
- ½ cup neroli hydrosol
- ½ cup rose geranium hydrosol
- 1 teaspoon jojoba oil
- 20 drops geranium essential oil
- 20 drops neroli essential oil

Try substituting lavender, lavandin, or rose hydrosol (or even plain distilled or purified water) for neroli or rose geranium hydrosol. You may also substitute lavender essential oil for neroli essential oil.

TO MAKE

Combine all the ingredients in a 16-ounce plastic or glass bottle. Shake well to blend. Pour into smaller storage container(s), preferably plastic squeeze bottles, if desired. Label and date.

TO STORE

No refrigeration is required, but for maximum freshness and potency, please use within 1 year. Store in a dark, cool cabinet or in the shower.

TO APPLY

Shake well before each use. Moisten your face with warm water. Using a damp, soft cloth, a cleansing pad, or your fingers, apply approximately 1 teaspoon over your entire face and throat (or more as necessary for use on the rest of your body). Rinse with warm water.

Use daily. Follow with astringent or toner.

MINT-LOVER'S WASH

Like the previous recipe, this one also dilutes the castile soap by 50 percent, but it uses distilled or purified water and subtly fragrant, mildly anti-inflammatory lemon balm hydrosol to create a very gentle liquid soap product for virtually all skin types. It is perfect for mint lovers and for those who insist on using soap and makes an effective, invigorating, aromatic, pick-me-up cleanser for the entire body.

YIELD: 2 cups

PREP TIME: 10 minutes

1 (8-ounce) bottle unscented liquid castile soap

1/2 cup lemon balm hydrosol

1/2 cup distilled or purified water

1 teaspoon jojoba oil

10–15 drops peppermint essential oil

10–15 drops spearmint essential oil

Try substituting another 1/2 cup of distilled or purified water for the lemon balm hydrosol if it is unavailable.

TO MAKE

Combine all the ingredients in a 16-ounce plastic or glass bottle. Shake well to blend. Pour into smaller storage container(s), preferably plastic squeeze bottles, if desired. Label and date.

TO STORE

No refrigeration is required, but for maximum freshness and potency, please use within 1 year. Store in a dark, cool cabinet or in the shower.

TO APPLY

Shake well before each use. Moisten skin with warm water. Using a damp, soft cloth, cleansing pad, or your fingers, apply approximately 1 teaspoon over your entire face and throat (or more as necessary for use on the body). Rinse with warm water.

Use daily. Follow with astringent or toner.

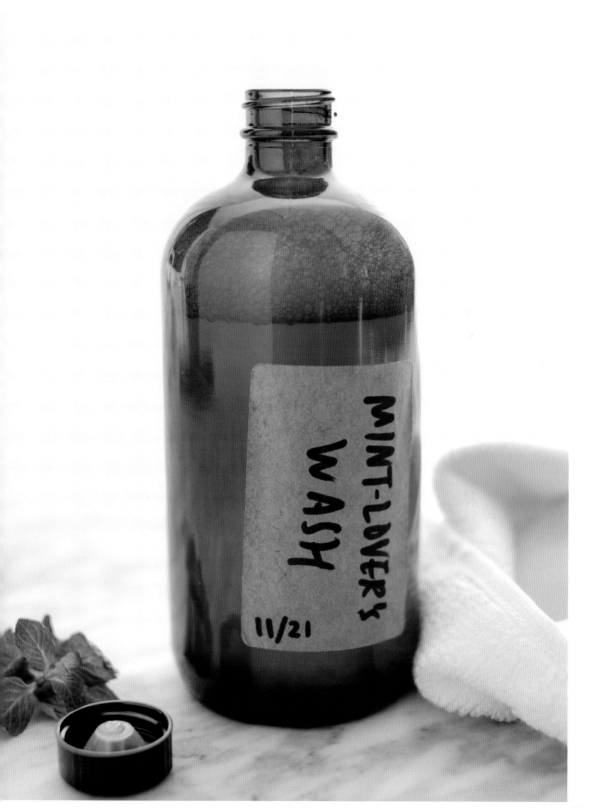

MINT-LOVER's WASH

11/21

REJUVENATING CLEANSING OIL

YIELD: 1/2 cup

PREP TIME: 10 to 15 minutes

This unique oil blend nourishes dry, parched skin and maintains the glow of normal, healthy skin. Oily skin can benefit from the vitamin- and mineral-rich oils, too, but make sure to apply the appropriate astringent following cleansing to remove any oil residue. This product is an excellent makeup remover, but follow with a second cleansing using this oil or another cleanser of your choice to ensure that your skin is deep-down clean. You can also use this oil as a massage or bath oil, or as "skin food" for normal and dry skin (applied before bedtime, preferably on damp skin, and left on overnight in lieu of regular moisturizer).

2   tablespoons almond or apricot kernel oil

2   tablespoons avocado or sunflower seed oil

2   tablespoons extra-virgin olive oil

2   tablespoons jojoba oil

2   capsules 200 IU vitamin E oil

20 drops sweet orange, grapefruit, lavender, frankincense (CO_2), or rosemary (ct. verbenon) essential oil

Including an essential oil is optional, but it adds a hint of fragrance and rejuvenating, skin-conditioning properties.

TO MAKE

Combine the almond, avocado, olive, and jojoba oils in your storage container; a plastic squeeze or pump bottle works great. Shake well to blend. Add the vitamin E oil capsules (pierce the capsule skin and squeeze the contents into the mix), then add the essential oil (if desired) and shake again. Label and date.

TO STORE

No refrigeration is required, but for maximum freshness and potency, please use within 6 months. Store in a dark, cool cabinet.

TO APPLY

Shake well before each use. Using a soft, damp cloth, a cleansing pad, or your fingers, apply approximately $^1\!/_2$ to 1 teaspoon over your entire face and throat. Massage for a minute. Rinse with warm water.

If you're using this blend as a bath oil, use 1 tablespoon per tubful of water.

Use daily. Follow with astringent or toner.

ALOE and HERBS CLEANSING CREAM

YIELD: 2 cups

PREP TIME: 30 minutes, plus 30 minutes to cool and set up

This ultra-rich cleansing cream removes makeup, dirt, and grime and has powerful moisturizing, hydrating, and anti-inflammatory properties. It's soothing to damaged and irritated skin and doubles as a fabulous face and body cream and after-sun rejuvenating remedy. If you're using it as a facial moisturizer, you'll need only a pea-size dollop. Use it as needed for your body.

½ cup almond, sunflower, apricot kernel, or jojoba oil

4 tablespoons unrefined coconut oil

3 tablespoons shea butter (refined or unrefined)

1 tablespoon beeswax or vegetable emulsifying wax

1 tablespoon cocoa butter

⅓ cup commercial aloe vera juice

¾ cup strong calendula blossom or chamomile flower tea

1 teaspoon vegetable glycerin

10 capsules 200 IU vitamin E oil

16 drops lavender essential oil

16 drops frankincense (CO_2), geranium, or rosemary (ct. verbenon) essential oil

8 drops calendula essential oil (CO_2) (optional)

Try substituting your favorite hydrosol or distilled or purified water for the calendula blossom or chamomile flower tea. If rosemary, frankincense, or geranium essential oils are unavailable, instead use an additional 16 drops of lavender essential oil.

TO MAKE

Following the Making Creams and Lotions technique on page 58, heat the almond oil, coconut oil, shea butter, beeswax, and cocoa butter until just melted. In another pan, warm the aloe vera juice, tea, and vegetable glycerin. Remove both pans from the heat. Pour the oil/butter/wax mixture into a blender and allow it to cool for approximately 20 minutes, or until it begins to turn slightly opaque.

Place the lid on the blender and remove the lid's plastic piece. With the blender turned on at medium speed, slowly drizzle the aloe juice/tea/glycerin mixture into the vortex of swirling fats below. Almost immediately the cream will turn off-white to very pale yellow and will begin to thicken. Blend for 10 to 15 seconds, or until all the watery mixture has been added, then check the consistency of the cream. It should have a smooth, glossy texture.

Turn off the blender and add the vitamin E oil and essential oils. Blend for another 5 seconds or so, until the cream is smooth and thick.

TO STORE

The cream will keep best in a dark, cool cabinet. Use within 60 to 90 days. If your storage area is very warm, please use the cream within 4 weeks for maximum freshness and potency. On the day that you notice any mold growing in your container, toss it out and make a fresh batch.

TO APPLY

Using a soft, damp cloth, a cleansing pad, or your fingers, apply approximately 1/2 to 1 teaspoon over your entire face and throat. Massage for a minute. Rinse off with warm water. Because this cream is very concentrated, a small amount goes a long way. Repeat if necessary, especially if you are wearing heavy foundation makeup or your skin is particularly dirty.

Use daily. Follow with astringent or toner.

LEMONY WHIP CLEANSING CREAM

YIELD: 2 cups

PREP TIME: 30 minutes, plus 30 minutes to cool and set up

Yes, you can use an oil-based cleansing cream to cleanse oily and combination skin. The oils in the cream will actually dissolve and break down the dirty oils and makeup on your skin. In this case, like removes like! If you feel that your skin needs additional cleansing, follow with a second application using this same product or another gentle cleanser of your choice.

½ cup apricot kernel, hazelnut, or jojoba oil

6 tablespoons unrefined coconut oil

2 tablespoons shea butter (refined or unrefined)

1 tablespoon beeswax or vegetable emulsifying wax

1 cup lemon balm hydrosol or distilled or purified water

1 teaspoon vegetable glycerin

10 capsules 200 IU vitamin E oil

20 drops lemon essential oil

10 drops grapefruit essential oil

10 drops sweet orange essential oil

TO MAKE

Following the Making Creams and Lotions technique on page 58, heat the apricot kernel oil, coconut oil, shea butter, and beeswax until just melted. In another pan, warm the hydrosol and vegetable glycerin, stirring gently. Remove both pans from the heat. Pour the oil/butter/wax mixture into a blender and allow it to cool for approximately 20 minutes, or until it begins to turn slightly opaque.

Place the lid on the blender and remove the lid's plastic piece. With the blender turned on at medium speed, slowly drizzle the hydrosol and glycerin mixture into the vortex of swirling fats below. Almost immediately the cream will turn off-white to very pale yellow and will begin to thicken. Blend for 10 to 15 seconds, or until all the watery mixture has been added, then check the consistency of the cream. It should have a smooth, glossy texture.

Turn off the blender and add the vitamin E oil and essential oils. Blend for another 5 seconds or so, until the cream is smooth and thick.

TO STORE

The cream will keep best in a dark, cool cabinet. Use within 60 to 90 days. If your storage area is very warm, please use the cream within 4 weeks for maximum freshness and potency. On the day that you notice any mold growing in your container, toss it out and make a fresh batch.

TO APPLY

Using a soft, damp cloth, a cleansing pad, or your fingers, apply approximately $\frac{1}{2}$ to 1 teaspoon of the cream over your entire face and throat. Massage for a minute. Rinse with warm water. Because this cream is very concentrated, a small amount goes a long way. Repeat if necessary, especially if you are wearing heavy foundation makeup or your skin is particularly dirty.

Use daily. Follow with astringent or toner.

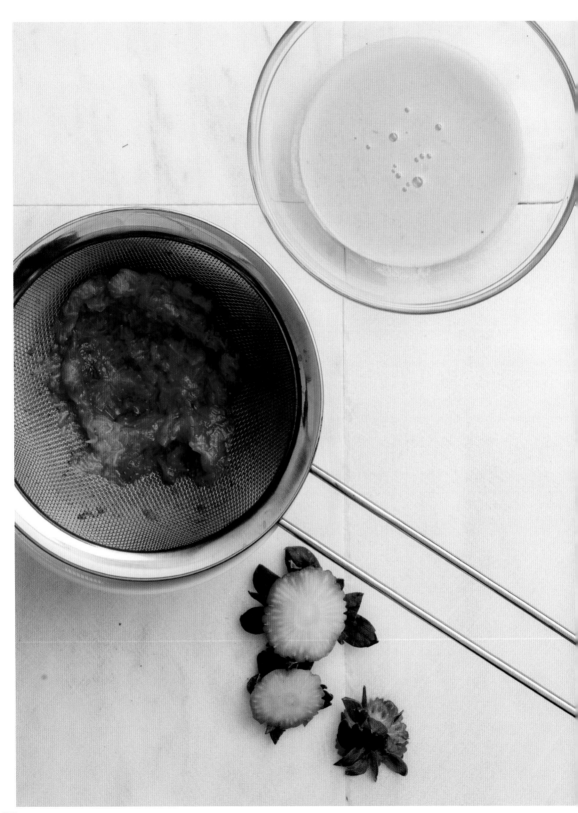

SKIN-SOFTENING STRAWBERRY CLEANSER

**SKIN TYPES
RECOMMENDED FOR**
normal
oily or acneic
combination

Pleasingly fragrant strawberry juice has gentle astringent and brightening properties, and plain yogurt has naturally occurring lactic acid. The combination creates an excellent exfoliating cleanser that will leave skin smooth and silky soft. This product is best used as a light cleanser for those who do not wear makeup. It does not store well, so please mix as needed.

YIELD: 1 application

PREP TIME: 5 to 10 minutes

4 very ripe medium strawberries, sliced, with green stems removed

1 teaspoon plain yogurt

TO MAKE

Thoroughly mash the strawberries in a small bowl with a fork or with a mortar and pestle. Press the resulting pulp through a mesh strainer or squeeze it through cheesecloth, muslin fabric, or a nylon stocking, catching the juice in a small bowl. Add the plain yogurt to the juice and stir to blend.

TO APPLY

Avoiding the eye area, apply the mixture to your face and neck and massage with your fingertips for a minute. Rinse with cool water.

Use daily when fresh strawberries are in season. Follow with astringent or toner.

Note: Because both strawberries and yogurt contain natural exfoliating acids, you may experience a slight stinging sensation. This is completely normal.

Astringents and Toners

Astringents and toners are water-based agents used to remove cleanser residue, balance pH, and hydrate the skin. They are also effective at removing excess perspiration and oil.

Astringents tend to be stronger than toners and are usually used on oily, combination, and normal skin types. Many commercial astringents contain isopropyl alcohol and/or acetone (a strong synthetic solvent found in nail polish removers), which are very drying and damaging to the skin. Herbal astringents, however, are gentle.

Toners perform the same function as astringents but are designed for normal, dry, sensitive, dehydrated, mature, and environmentally damaged skin.

Always apply astringents and toners to the face and neck with a 100 percent cotton ball or pad using upward and outward strokes.

Remember that aromatic hydrosols (page 224) on their own make good toners and gentle astringents. As a bonus, hydrosols do not require refrigeration.

Storage Tips

A handful of the following astringent and toner recipes require refrigeration and should be used within 1 to 2 weeks for maximum freshness. Please read the recipe directions carefully so as to avoid spoilage of your fresh-made product. Whether or not they are refrigerated, store your products in tightly sealed and labeled bottles or spritzers.

REFRESHING ASTRINGENT

SKIN TYPES RECOMMENDED FOR
normal
oily or acneic
combination

This product is wonderful to use chilled in the warmer months. It has a cooling, fresh fragrance and can also be used as an aftershave on the face or applied to the legs, underarms, or bikini line (as tolerated; it will sting a bit) after shaving to prevent ingrown hairs.

YIELD: 1 cup

PREP TIME: 2 weeks, plus 5 minutes to strain and bottle

- 2 tablespoons dried peppermint, spearmint, or lemon balm leaves or 4 tablespoons fresh, chopped
- 1/2 cup plain vodka
- 1/2 cup witch hazel
- 12 drops peppermint or spearmint essential oil

TO MAKE

Combine the herbs with the vodka, witch hazel, and essential oil in a half-pint glass jar. Screw on the lid and label and date the jar. Set in a dark, cool cabinet to steep for 2 weeks, shaking the jar vigorously every day.

After 2 weeks, strain the liquid through a fine strainer lined with cheesecloth, muslin, or a coffee filter to remove all particulate matter. Pour into an 8-ounce storage container. Label and date.

TO STORE

No refrigeration is required, but for maximum freshness and potency, please use within 6 months. Store in a dark, cool cabinet.

TO APPLY

Shake well before each application. Saturate a cotton ball or pad and apply the astringent to the face, neck, chest, shoulders, or back. Avoid the eye area.

Use daily. Follow with light moisturizer.

**SKIN TYPES
RECOMMENDED FOR**

normal

oily

combination

oily mature

LEMON REFRESHER

The tart, lemony aroma of this astringent is refreshing and stimulating. Try chilling it to use on a hot summer day. Avoid using it on sensitive, dehydrated, environmentally damaged, sunburned, windburned, or irritated skin.

YIELD: 1/2 cup

PREP TIME: 5 to 10 minutes

1/2   cup witch hazel

Juice of 1/2 medium lemon

2   drops lemon essential oil (optional)

TO MAKE

Combine all the ingredients in a 4-ounce plastic or glass bottle and shake well to blend. Label and date.

TO STORE

No refrigeration is required, but please use within 1 to 2 weeks, then discard. Store in a dark, cool cabinet.

TO APPLY

Shake well before each application. Saturate a cotton ball or pad and apply the astringent onto the face, neck, shoulders, chest, or back. You can apply this astringent throughout the day as a refresher. Avoid the eye area.

Use daily. Follow with light moisturizer.

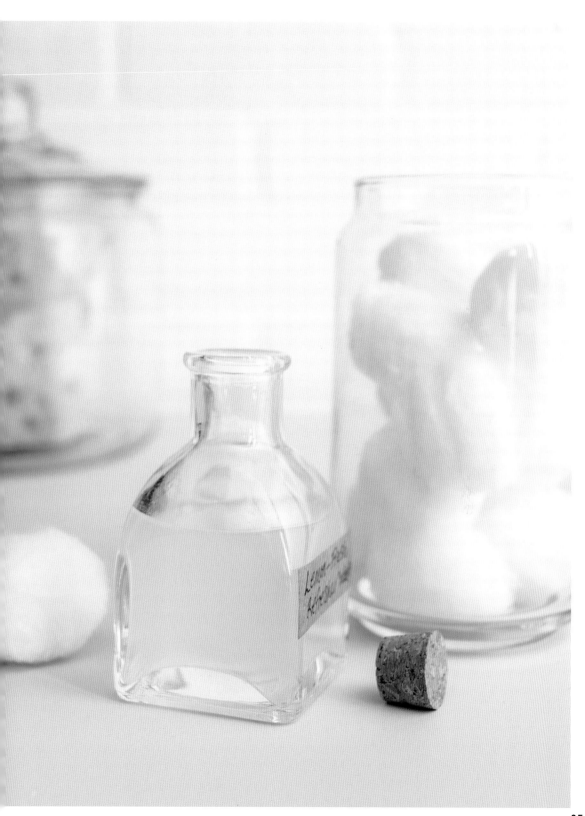

GREASE-BE-GONE PARSLEY and PEPPERMINT ASTRINGENT

YIELD: 2 cups

PREP TIME: 35 minutes

This strong, green herbal infusion makes a gentle yet powerful astringent to use on those days when your skin feels particularly hot and greasy. It effectively removes excess oil without causing dryness and is wonderful for use during hot flashes.

- 2 cups distilled or purified water
- 1/4 cup chopped fresh parsley or 2 tablespoons dried
- 1/4 cup chopped fresh peppermint or 2 tablespoons dried
- 6 drops peppermint essential oil (optional)

TO MAKE

In a small saucepan, bring the water to a boil and then remove from the heat. Add the herbs, cover, and allow to steep for 30 minutes. Pour through a strainer lined with cheesecloth, muslin, or a coffee filter to remove all particulate matter. Add the essential oil (if desired) and stir to blend. Pour into storage container(s). Shake well. Label and date.

TO STORE

Refrigerate for up to 1 week, then discard.

TO APPLY

Shake well before each application. Saturate a cotton ball or pad and apply the astringent to the face, neck, shoulders, chest, or back. Avoid the eye area.

Use daily. Follow with light moisturizer.

BALANCE RESTORER

When your skin maintains the correct pH, it has a much better chance of fighting off dryness and infections. The vinegar in this astringent helps combat the alkaline residue that soap and other cleansers can leave behind, helping to balance your skin's pH and soften the skin. It doubles as a hair product, effectively removing styling product buildup and enhancing shine. Simply pour the entire recipe over your hair after rinsing out conditioner. You can use this product weekly on your hair, if desired.

YIELD: 2 cups

PREP TIME: 5 to 10 minutes

1³⁄4 cups distilled or purified water

1⁄4 cup raw apple cider vinegar

10 drops essential oil*

*Try using frankincense (CO_2), geranium, lavender, or rosemary (ct. verbenon) essential oil(s), singly or in combination.

TO MAKE

Combine all the ingredients in a 16-ounce plastic or glass bottle. Shake well to blend. Pour into storage container(s). Label and date.

TO STORE

No refrigeration is required, but for maximum freshness and potency, please use within 1 year. Store in a dark, cool cabinet.

TO APPLY

Shake well before each application. Saturate a cotton ball or pad and apply the astringent to the face, neck, shoulders, chest, or back. It also makes a terrific body splash for comforting itchy skin. Avoid the eye area.

Use daily. Follow with moisturizer.

ACNE-SOOTHING ASTRINGENT

YIELD: 2 cups

PREP TIME: 35 minutes

This remedial astringent is particularly soothing for active, weeping acne, but it is also effective for oily, combination, and normal skin suffering from excessive oiliness and breakouts. It doubles as a skin-mending wash for minor cuts and abrasions and also works well as a hair rinse if your scalp is oily.

- 2 cups distilled or purified water
- 1 tablespoon dried calendula or chamomile flowers or 2 tablespoons fresh, chopped
- 1 tablespoon dried yarrow flowers or 2 tablespoons fresh, chopped
- 6 drops juniper, rosemary (ct. verbenon), lemongrass, or peppermint essential oil

TO MAKE

In a small saucepan, bring the water to a boil and then remove from the heat. Add the herbs, cover, and let steep for 30 minutes. Pour through a fine strainer lined with cheesecloth, muslin, or a coffee filter to remove all particulate matter. Add the essential oil and stir to blend. Pour into storage container(s). Shake well. Label and date.

TO STORE

Refrigerate for up to 1 week, then discard.

TO APPLY

Shake well before each application. Saturate a cotton ball or pad and apply the astringent to the face, neck, chest, shoulders, or back. Avoid the eye area.

Use daily. Follow with light moisturizer.

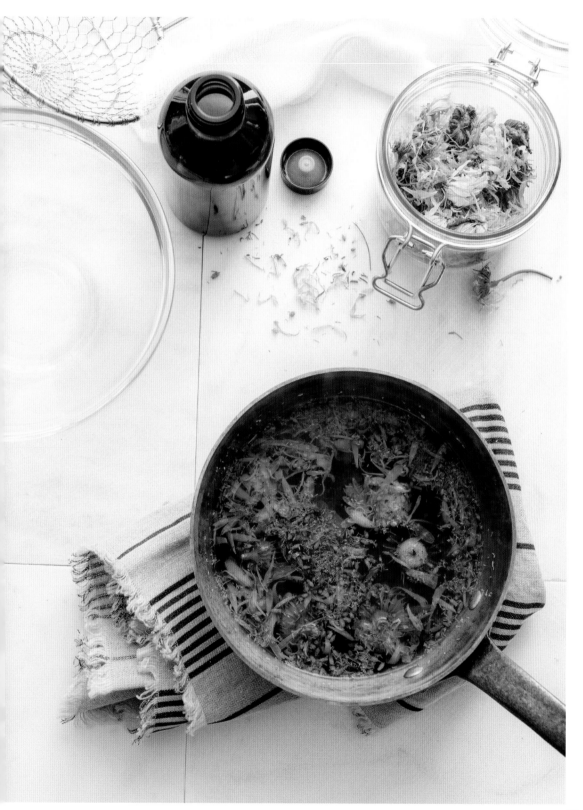

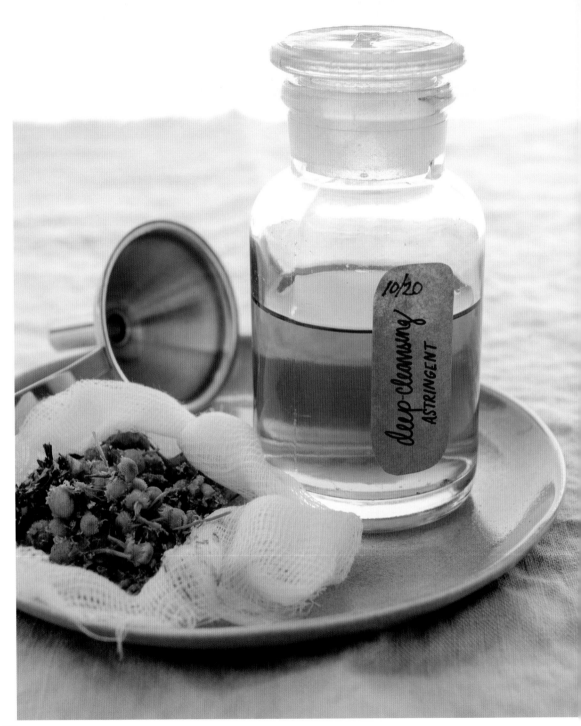

DEEP-CLEANSING ASTRINGENT

SKIN TYPES RECOMMENDED FOR

normal

oily or acneic

combination

This astringent is actually an herbal tincture, or alcohol extract, for topical application. It is one of my more potent formulations for thoroughly removing excess oil and perspiration without overdrying the skin. Use it after doing anything that causes you to sweat profusely.

YIELD: 2 cups

PREP TIME: 2 weeks, plus 5 minutes to strain and bottle

- 2 cups plain vodka
- 1 tablespoon dried chamomile flowers or 2 tablespoons fresh, chopped
- 1 tablespoon dried lemon balm leaves or 2 tablespoons fresh, chopped
- 1 tablespoon dried pepper-mint leaves or 2 tablespoons fresh, chopped
- 1 tablespoon dried rosemary leaves or 2 tablespoons fresh, chopped
- 1 tablespoon dried sage leaves or 2 tablespoons fresh, chopped
- 1 tablespoon dried strawberry leaves or 2 tablespoons fresh, chopped
- 1 tablespoon dried yarrow flowers or 2 tablespoons fresh, chopped

TO MAKE

Combine all the ingredients in a 1-pint glass jar. Screw on the lid and label and date the jar. Set in a dark, cool cabinet to steep for 2 weeks, shaking the jar vigorously every day.

After 2 weeks, strain the liquid through a fine strainer lined with cheese-cloth, muslin, or a coffee filter to remove all particulate matter. Pour into storage container(s). Label and date.

TO STORE

No refrigeration is required, but for maximum freshness and potency, please use within 2 years. Store in a dark, cool cabinet.

TO APPLY

Shake before each application. Saturate a cotton ball and apply the astringent to the face, neck, chest, shoulders, or back. Avoid the eye area.

Use daily. Follow with light moisturizer.

SPICY AFTERSHAVE TONIC

YIELD: 2 cups

PREP TIME: 2 weeks, plus 10 minutes to strain and bottle

This aftershave tonic smells delightfully spicy. When strained, it can also be used as a scented hair rinse or scalp cleanser for oily or normal hair. Avoid use on blond or bleached hair, as it may temporarily stain.

1 cup plain vodka

1 cup witch hazel

1 sprig fresh peppermint or spearmint

1 sprig fresh rosemary

1 cinnamon stick

10 whole cloves

Peel of 1 medium lemon, cut into thin strips

Peel of 1 medium orange, cut into thin strips

1 teaspoon vegetable glycerin

10 drops sweet orange or cardamom essential oil

TO MAKE

Combine all the ingredients in a 1-pint or slightly larger jar. Screw on the lid and label and date the jar. Set in a dark, cool cabinet to steep for 2 weeks, shaking the jar vigorously every day.

After 2 weeks, strain the liquid through a fine strainer lined with cheesecloth, muslin, or a coffee filter to remove all particulate matter. Pour into storage container(s). (You can add fresh citrus peels or spices to the storage containers for aesthetic appeal if desired.) Label and date.

TO STORE

No refrigeration is required, but for maximum freshness and potency, please use within 6 months. Store in a dark, cool cabinet.

TO APPLY

Shake well before each application. Saturate a cotton ball or pad, and apply to your face and neck after each shave, or just splash some on with your hands. To help prevent ingrown hairs, apply the tonic similarly to any other area you might shave — legs, underarms, bikini area, and so on. Be aware, it will sting a bit!

Use daily. Follow with moisturizer.

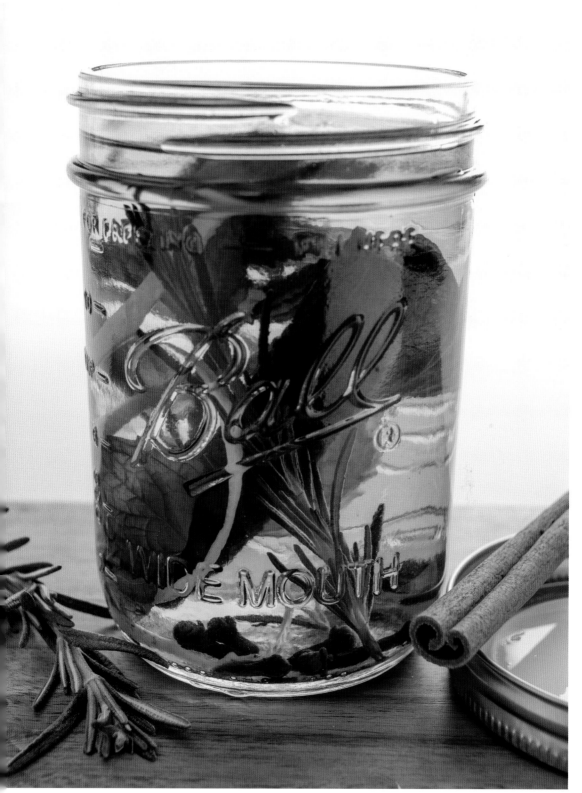

TRANQUILITY TONER

This is a very gentle toner suitable for most skin types and anyone who loves the subtly sweet, relaxing aroma of lavender.

YIELD: 1 cup

PREP TIME: 2 weeks, plus 5 minutes to strain and bottle

$1/4$ cup dried lavender buds or $1/3$ cup fresh

1 cup witch hazel

$1/2$ teaspoon vegetable glycerin

12 drops lavender essential oil

TO MAKE

Combine the lavender buds and witch hazel in a half-pint glass jar. Screw on the lid and label and date the jar. Set in a dark, cool cabinet to steep for 2 weeks, shaking the jar vigorously every day.

After 2 weeks, strain the liquid through a fine strainer lined with cheesecloth, muslin, or a coffee filter to remove all particulate matter. Add the vegetable glycerin and essential oil and stir to blend. Pour into an 8-ounce storage container. Label and date.

TO STORE

No refrigeration is required, but for maximum freshness and potency, please use within 6 months. Store in a dark, cool cabinet.

TO APPLY

Shake well before each application. Saturate a cotton ball or pad and apply toner to the face, neck, chest, shoulders, or back. If you're using it as a body splash, be generous with application — it feels and smells so good! Avoid the eye area.

Use daily. Follow with light moisturizer.

MOISTURE INFUSION TONIC

SKIN TYPES RECOMMENDED FOR
all

YIELD: 2 cups

PREP TIME: 1^{1}/2 hours, plus 5 minutes to strain and bottle

Comfrey and marshmallow roots produce a soothing mucilage that has wonderful comforting and hydrating properties for all skin types, including the tender skin of infants and the elderly. This tonic is especially beneficial for those with dehydrated, sensitive, sunburned, windburned, mature, or environmentally damaged skin. Try using it as a body splash in winter, when skin tends to be severely dry.

- 2 cups distilled or purified water

- 1 tablespoon chopped, dried comfrey root or 3 tablespoons fresh, chopped

- 1 tablespoon chopped dried marshmallow root or 3 tablespoons fresh, chopped

TO MAKE

In a small saucepan, bring the water to a boil, then reduce the heat to the lowest setting, add the herbs, cover, and let simmer gently for 30 minutes. Remove from the heat and let cool for 1 hour.

Pour the liquid through a strainer, mashing the root bits as best you can with the back of a spoon to completely extract the gooey, slippery mucilage. Pour the liquid into storage container(s). Label and date.

Recipe continues on next page

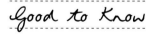

Good to Know

SIMMERING VS. STEEPING

Because roots are tougher than leaves and flowers, they require a period of gentle cooking or decocting — instead of merely steeping in hot water — to extract their beneficial components.

**Moisture Infusion
Tonic** *continued*

TO STORE

Refrigerate for up to 1 week, then discard.

TO APPLY

Shake well before each application. Saturate a cotton ball or pad and apply toner to your face and neck. If you're using it as a hydrating body splash, be generous with application.

Use daily. Follow with moisturizer.

DELICATE ELDER FLOWER TONER

This calming tonic is so gentle that it can even be used on infants. It is wonderful for soothing diaper rash, eczema, and dermatitis. Anyone with sensitive, dry, mature, dehydrated, sunburned, windburned, mature, or environmentally damaged skin will especially benefit from the hydrating properties of this toner.

SKIN TYPES RECOMMENDED FOR
all

YIELD: 1 cup

PREP TIME: 45 minutes, plus 5 minutes to strain and bottle

- 1 cup distilled or purified water
- 1 tablespoon dried elder flowers or 2 tablespoons fresh
- 1 teaspoon vegetable glycerin
- 8 drops lavender essential oil (optional)

TO MAKE

In a small saucepan, bring the water to a boil, then remove from the heat, add the elder flowers, cover, and let steep for 45 minutes.

Strain through a fine strainer lined with cheesecloth, muslin, or a coffee filter to remove all particulate matter. Pour into an 8-ounce storage container. Add the glycerin and the essential oil (if desired) and shake vigorously to blend. Label and date.

TO STORE

Refrigerate for up to 1 week, then discard.

TO APPLY

Shake well before each application. Saturate a cotton ball or pad and apply toner to the face, neck, chest, shoulders, or back. It may also be used as a soothing body splash. Avoid the eye area.

Use daily. Follow with moisturizer.

THYME *to* HEAL TONIC

YIELD: 1 cup

PREP TIME: 2 weeks, plus 5 minutes to strain and bottle

This recipe combines a thyme tincture with tea tree essential oil. The resultant formula has astringent, antibacterial, antifungal, and antiviral properties and is a useful sanitizer when you are living with or working around people who have a cold or the flu. Decant a portion of it into a small plastic spritzer bottle, and keep it with you at all times so that you can spray it periodically on your hands and face, your phone, the handle of your grocery cart, and anything else you want to disinfect. Spraying it directly into the air will help purify the surrounding environment.

It also works as an effective remedy for active or weeping acne, boils, cuts, scrapes, bug bites, and other skin irritations. Just apply it several times per day until the irritation or infection clears up. If you have oily or combination skin, you can use it as a facial astringent.

Note: Due to the alcohol content, this tonic may sting when you apply it to open skin.

1 cup plain vodka

¼ cup dried thyme leaves or ½ cup fresh, chopped

24 drops tea tree essential oil

TO MAKE

Combine all the ingredients in a half-pint or slightly larger jar. Screw on the lid and label and date the jar. Set in a cool, dark cabinet to steep for 2 weeks, shaking the jar vigorously every day.

After 2 weeks, pour the liquid through a strainer lined with cheesecloth, muslin, or a coffee filter to remove all particulate matter. Pour into an 8-ounce storage container or several smaller containers. Label and date.

TO STORE

No refrigeration is required, but for maximum freshness and potency, please use within 2 years.

TO APPLY

Shake well before each application. Saturate a cotton ball or pad and apply tonic to face, throat, chest, shoulders, or back or to other parts of the body affected by irritations or minor-to-moderate infections. Avoid the eye area.

Use daily or as needed. Follow with moisturizer.

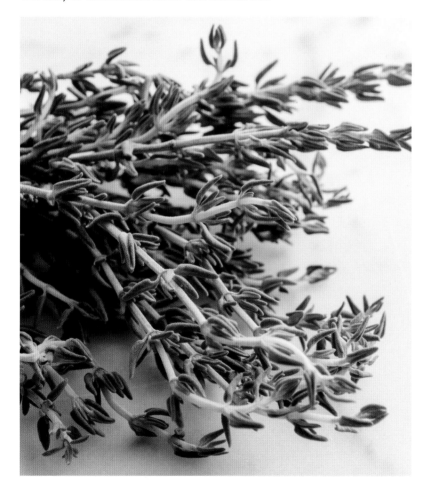

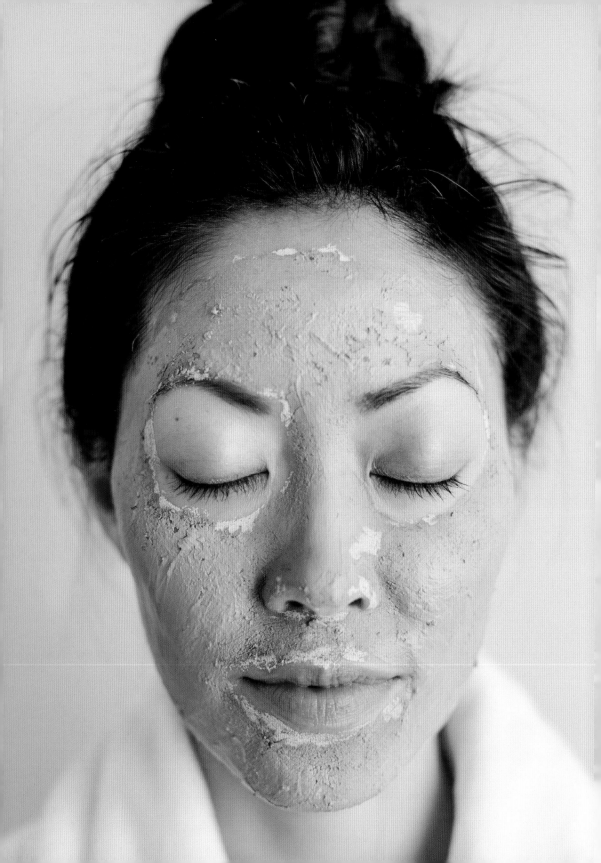

Chapter 5

REVIVE

Recipes for Masks, Steams, and Scrubs

The following recipes perform a deeper cleansing of your skin than the ones offered in chapter 4. They aid in removing toxins and accumulations of surface dead skin cells while simultaneously improving circulation. Some even tone and tighten; calm inflammation; and brighten, hydrate, and soften the skin. If you have sensitive, mature, or environmentally damaged skin, be sure to read the contraindications for each type of product carefully. Even though all of my formulas are gentle and nourishing, some may still irritate extremely sensitive skin.

Masks

Masks for the beautification and purification of both the face and body date back to ancient civilizations. Clay was especially valued in masks for its ability to absorb animal, mineral, and botanical dyes and its use as body paint during important rituals and events.

Today, though, masks are used primarily for cosmetic purposes to deep-clean the skin. Depending on their ingredients, masks can increase circulation, remove toxins, tone and tighten, act as nonabrasive exfoliants, hydrate and moisturize, calm inflammation, and soften the skin. Masks can be made from myriad natural ingredients such as clay or finely ground grains, which absorb excess oil and physically slough dead cells from the skin's surface and stimulate a sluggish complexion. Masks can also be made from such succulent ingredients as honey, cream, and fresh, ripe peaches and bananas; all of these ingredients moisturize and bring a glow to your complexion. Masks containing acidic ingredients such as papaya, pineapple, raspberries, yogurt, or buttermilk serve as gentle, natural chemical exfoliants that leave skin velvety smooth and deeply hydrated.

Application Tips

Before applying any of these masks, be sure to pull your hair up off your face and neck — some of the juicier masks have a habit of trickling down a bit into places where they're not welcome. A mask should always be applied to freshly cleansed, barely damp skin. For specific application tips and times, see individual recipes.

Everyone's BASIC CLAY MASK

SKIN TYPES RECOMMENDED FOR
all

All clay masks gently exfoliate as they tighten, stimulate circulation, remineralize, and soften the skin. This mask can be customized according to skin type, making it gentle enough to be used by anyone. Mix this recipe as needed; do not store.

YIELD: 1 treatment

PREP TIME: 5 minutes

1 tablespoon powdered white cosmetic clay or kaolin

For dry skin: About 2 teaspoons heavy cream, half-and-half, or full-fat coconut milk

For normal skin: About 2 teaspoons low-fat or whole dairy milk, almond milk, or coconut water

For oily skin: About 2 teaspoons purified water or commercial aloe vera juice

TO MAKE

In a very small bowl, use a spoon or tiny whisk to combine the clay with enough of the liquid of your choice to form a smooth, spreadable paste.

TO APPLY

Using your fingers, spread the paste onto your face and neck. Let dry completely, which should take 20 to 30 minutes, preferably while you are lying down. The mask will feel like it is lifting and tightening your skin. When you're ready, rinse off with warm water.

Use one or two times per week. Follow with moisturizer.

Good to Know

CLAY MASKS MAKE GREAT OVERNIGHT PIMPLE REMEDIES

With a cotton swab apply a dab of any of my three clay masks to each pimple and leave on while you sleep. In the morning, rinse off the remaining bits of mask with warm water. The clay absorbs excess oil during the night and aids in drying out blemishes.

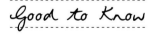

GREEN GODDESS PURIFYING CLAY MASK

YIELD: 1 treatment

PREP TIME: 5 minutes

Due to its gentleness, this mask is my preferred method of exfoliation for acneic skin. (Most granular, enzyme, and fruit-acid masks can be quite irritating to acneic skin.) French green clay combined with anti-inflammatory essential oils is very beneficial for cystic and weeping or active acne conditions that are also sensitive. It aids in removing impurities and toxins from beneath the surface of the skin. You can also apply this drying mask to chest or back areas that have blemishes. Mix this recipe as needed; do not store.

1   tablespoon powdered French green clay

    About 2 teaspoons commercial aloe vera juice, strong peppermint tea, or water

2   drops German chamomile, helichrysum, or lavender essential oil

TO MAKE

In a very small bowl, use a spoon or tiny whisk to combine the clay with enough aloe vera juice to form a smooth, spreadable paste. Stir in the essential oil.

TO APPLY

Using your fingers, spread the paste onto your face and neck. Let dry completely, which should take 20 to 30 minutes, preferably while you are lying down. The mask will feel like it is lifting and tightening your skin. When you're ready, rinse off with warm water.

Use one or two times per week. Follow with light moisturizer.

If your chest or back is blemished, make an additional batch and apply there as well.

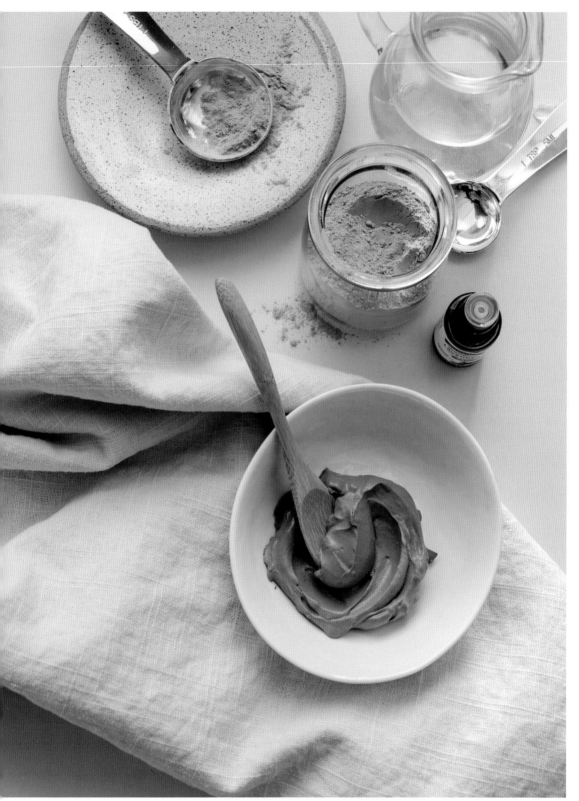

**SKIN TYPES
RECOMMENDED FOR**
normal
oily or acneic
combination
oily-to-normal mature

YIELD: 1 treatment

PREP TIME: 5 minutes

ROSY RED BALANCING CLAY MASK

This mask is subtly fragrant, tightening, lifting, mineralizing, sebum-balancing, and quite soothing to irritated skin. If your skin is sensitive and/or environmentally damaged, you can still partake of the benefits of this mask, but only leave it on for 10 minutes so that it doesn't become too tight and drying. Mix this recipe as needed; do not store.

1 tablespoon powdered red clay

About 2 teaspoons neroli, rose, or rose geranium hydrosol or water

2 drops geranium, lavender, neroli, or rose otto essential oil

TO MAKE

In a very small bowl, use a spoon or tiny whisk to combine the clay with enough hydrosol to form a smooth, spreadable paste. Stir in the essential oil.

TO APPLY

Using your fingers, spread the paste onto your face and neck. Let dry completely, which should take 20 to 30 minutes, preferably while you are lying down. The mask will feel like it is lifting and tightening your skin. When you're ready, rinse off with warm water.

Use one or two times per week. Follow with moisturizer.

If your chest or back is blemished, make an additional batch and apply there as well.

YOGURT EXFOLIATING MASK

SKIN TYPES RECOMMENDED FOR
all, except very sensitive

Due to its lactic acid content, plain yogurt is a very gentle, soothing, and nonabrasive exfoliant. Its mild bleaching properties are great for evening out a fading tan or blotchy skin. The more often you use this mask, the more noticeable the benefits.

YIELD: 1 treatment

PREP TIME: 1 minute

1   tablespoon plain yogurt

TO APPLY

Using your fingers or a cosmetic fan brush, apply the yogurt to your face, neck, and chest (if desired). Then lie down with a towel wrapped around your hair and another under your neck, as the yogurt can become a bit runny when it reaches skin temperature. Relax for 20 to 30 minutes, then rinse off with warm water.

Use one or two times per week, or as desired. Follow with moisturizer.

*Avoid if your skin is
irritated, sunburned, or
windburned; use as tol-
erated on environmen-
tally damaged skin.*

YIELD: 1 treatment

PREP TIME: 10 to
15 minutes

NO-MORE-PORES DOUBLE MASK

The papaya and pineapple included in Mask 1 contain protein-dissolving enzymes that help lift away dry, scaly skin, which, over time, can build up on the surface and leave a dull appearance. The ingredients in Mask 2 will temporarily firm and tighten your skin. With repeated use, this mask duo will make your skin smoother, its tone more even, and your pores smaller and more refined (likely due to the removal of dead skin debris, which can clog and stretch the pore walls). The result? Skin glowing with healthy radiance! Mix this recipe as needed; do not store.

Note: If you have dry skin, you may want to apply a light moisturizer after Mask 1 and before Mask 2. If your skin is especially sensitive or irritated, skip Mask 2 and simply apply a teaspoon of aloe vera juice to your face and throat to cool and calm your skin.

Mask 1

¼ cup raw papaya

1 teaspoon fresh, raw pineapple juice (optional)

Mask 2

1 tablespoon powdered white cosmetic clay or kaolin

About 2 teaspoons strong peppermint, rosemary, or sage infusion (see Making an Herbal Infusion, page 212), or distilled or purified water

Recipe continues on next page

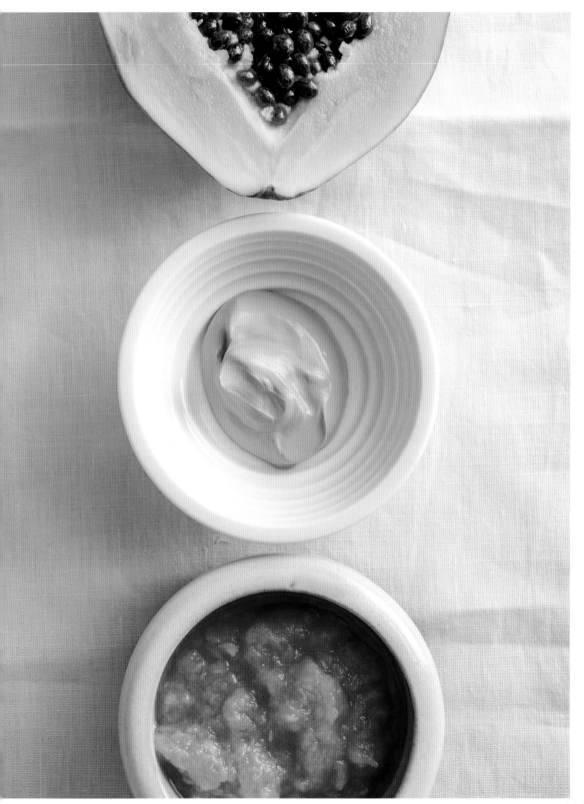

Mask 1

TO MAKE

Using a mortar and pestle or a small bowl and fork, mash the papaya and combine with the pineapple juice (if desired). The mashed fruit should have the consistency of a smooth paste.

TO APPLY

Using your fingers, gently pat this juicy pulp onto your face, neck, and chest (if desired). Then lie down with a towel wrapped around your hair and another under your neck, as the mashed fruit can be a bit runny. Relax for 15 to 20 minutes. Your skin will probably tingle, but that just means the natural fruit acids and enzymes are working. When you're finished, rinse off with warm water.

Use one time per week. Follow with Mask 2.

Mask 2

TO MAKE

In a very small bowl, use a spoon or tiny whisk to combine the clay with enough of the herbal infusion to form a smooth, spreadable paste.

TO APPLY

Using your fingers, spread the paste onto your face and neck. Let dry completely, which should take 20 to 30 minutes, preferably while you are lying down. When you're ready, rinse off with warm water.

Use one time per week. Follow with moisturizer.

SOOTHING *and* SOFTENING HONEY MASK

SKIN TYPES RECOMMENDED FOR
all

YIELD: 1 treatment

PREP TIME: 5 minutes

Honey acts as a humectant, drawing moisture from the air to the skin, which makes this mask deeply soothing and hydrating, especially for those with dry, sensitive, or environmentally damaged skin. It's wonderful to use during the cold, dry winter season, in areas of low humidity, and for people who do a great deal of traveling via airplane. Mix this recipe as needed; do not store.

- 1 tablespoon raw honey
- 1 teaspoon finely ground sunflower seed meal
- 1 teaspoon raw wheat germ

TO MAKE

Use a small whisk or spoon to thoroughly combine all the ingredients in a very small bowl. Let the mixture set for a couple of minutes to thicken a bit before applying it.

TO APPLY

Using your fingers, spread the honey mixture onto your face and neck. Then lie down with a towel wrapped around your hair and another under your neck. Relax for 30 minutes, then rinse off the mask with a warm, damp cloth. The honey will become thinner and somewhat runny as it warms to body temperature, so be sure to tuck your hair away from your face prior to application or you'll have a sticky mess.

Use as often as desired. Follow with moisturizer if necessary.

SWEET-*as*-HONEY MASSAGE MASK

YIELD: 1 treatment

PREP TIME: 1 minute

This is a delicious way to soften, deeply hydrate, and moisturize your skin. It also boosts circulation, which will leave your skin with a rosy glow. This mask is especially beneficial for those with dry, sunburned, windburned, mature, or environmentally damaged skin. Mix this recipe as needed; do not store.

2–3   teaspoons raw honey, at room temperature

TO APPLY

The honey will become thinner and somewhat runny as it warms to body temperature, so be sure to wear a shower cap or tuck your hair away from your face prior to application or you'll have a sticky mess.

Using your fingers, apply a very thin coat of honey to your entire face, neck, and chest (if desired). When the honey is spread evenly, it will bead on your skin much like water beads on your car after a rain shower. Lie down with a towel wrapped around your hair and another under your neck and rest for 15 minutes or so. Your skin will begin to feel warm and relaxed. Don't fall asleep!

Before rinsing, give yourself a circulation-boosting massage by patting your skin lightly with your fingertips in quick tapping motions, as though you were playing the piano, for 5 minutes. When you're ready, rinse off with a warm, damp cloth.

Use as desired. Follow with moisturizer if necessary.

APPLESAUCE *and* WHEAT GERM MOISTURIZING MASK

SKIN TYPES RECOMMENDED FOR
all, except oily and combination

This pampering mask leaves skin ultra-moisturized and is particularly soothing (especially if it is chilled) on hot, sunburned, or windburned skin. Mix this recipe as needed; do not store.

YIELD: 1 treatment

PREP TIME: 10 minutes

2 teaspoons applesauce

2 teaspoons raw wheat germ

$1/2$ teaspoon almond, apricot kernel, extra-virgin olive, jojoba, or sunflower oil

TO MAKE

Combine the applesauce and wheat germ in a very small bowl and use a small whisk or spoon to thoroughly mix. Allow the mixture to thicken for 5 minutes, or until the wheat germ absorbs some of the liquid. Have the oil ready to use after the mask application.

TO APPLY

Using your fingers, spread the mixture over your face and neck. Lie down with a towel wrapped around your hair and another under your neck. Relax and think pleasant thoughts while your skin drinks in all this nourishing moisture. After 20 to 30 minutes, rinse off with warm water.

Follow with a nourishing oil facial massage: apply the oil of your choice to your face and neck, and massage for 5 minutes using gentle, circular motions. Remove any excess oil by gently patting your skin with a tissue, or massage residual oil into your arms, knees, elbows, or other parts in need of softening. Your face will be moist, warm, and glowing.

Use as desired. Follow with moisturizer if necessary.

PEACHES and CREAM GLOW MASK

YIELD: 1 treatment

PREP TIME: 5 minutes

This mask is reminiscent of homemade peach ice cream — summery, sweet, and smooth — and it is as aromatic and delicious as it is nourishing and moisturizing for your skin. Try a spoonful or two before putting it on your skin. You may be tempted to mix up a larger batch, add a dab of honey, and drink it for lunch! Mix this recipe as needed; do not store.

½ very ripe small peach, peeled

1 tablespoon heavy cream or full-fat coconut milk

TO MAKE

Using a mortar and pestle or a small bowl and fork, mash the peach and combine with the cream until smooth.

TO APPLY

Using your fingers, spread the mixture over your face, neck, and chest (if desired). Lie down with a towel wrapped around your hair and another under your neck. Relax for 30 minutes, then rinse off with warm water.

Use as desired. Follow with moisturizer if necessary.

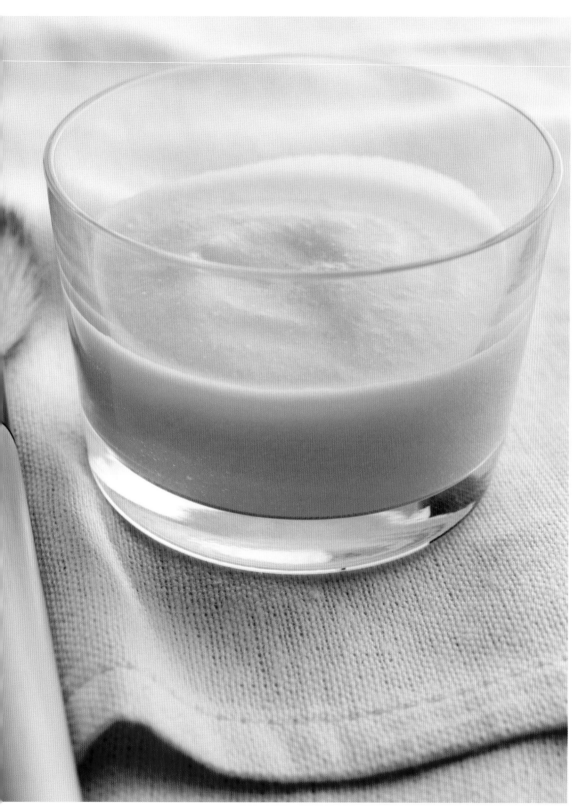

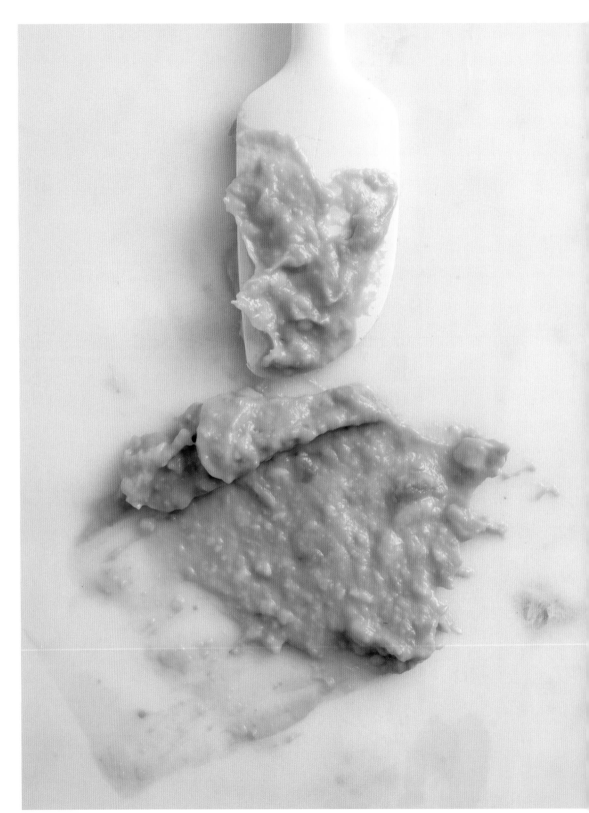

LUSCIOUSLY CREAMY AVOCADO and BUTTERMILK MASK

SKIN TYPES RECOMMENDED FOR
normal to very dry
mature

YIELD: 1 treatment

PREP TIME: 5 minutes

This incredibly nourishing and moisturizing mask leaves skin feeling velvety soft. The buttermilk gives it a slight bleaching effect that can help even out blotchy skin if used at least twice per week. This mask is especially beneficial for those with rough, chapped, or environmentally damaged skin. The mixture can also serve as a hair-conditioning treatment that is useful for normal, dry, frizzy, or chemically damaged hair. For use on hair, make a larger batch; apply to your hair, cover your head with plastic wrap or a shower cap, and leave on for 30 minutes, then rinse and lightly shampoo. Mix this recipe as needed; do not store.

¼   very ripe small avocado

About 1 tablespoon buttermilk

TO MAKE

Scoop out the avocado pulp and mash it, using a mortar and pestle or a small bowl and fork, and blend with just enough buttermilk to form a creamy paste.

TO APPLY

This mask can be a bit runny, so safeguard your hair and clothes prior to application. Using your fingers, apply the paste to your face, neck, and chest (if desired). Lie down with a towel wrapped around your hair and another under your neck. If possible, apply this mask in the early morning and lie in the early sun to allow the avocado oils to warm and penetrate your skin. Relax for 20 to 30 minutes, then rinse off with warm water.

Use as desired. Follow with moisturizer if necessary.

MELLOW YELLOW BANANA CREAM MASK

Bananas and cream will moisturize, hydrate, and pamper even the driest skin. Try to make this mask a healthy, yummy habit that your skin will relish. Should a bit of this delectably scrumptious mask drip into your mouth, it's fine to savor it! Mix this recipe as needed; do not store.

1 (2-inch) chunk very ripe banana

1–2 teaspoons cream (light or heavy) or full-fat coconut milk

TO MAKE

Using a mortar and pestle or a very small bowl and fork, mash the banana with just enough cream or coconut milk to make a smooth, spreadable paste.

TO APPLY

Using your fingers, spread the banana mixture onto your face, throat, and chest (if desired). Lie down with a towel wrapped around your hair and another under your neck. Relax for 20 to 30 minutes, then rinse off with warm water.

Use as desired. Follow with moisturizer if necessary.

EXFOLIATING OATMEAL MASK

SKIN TYPES RECOMMENDED FOR all, except very sensitive

Avoid if your skin is sunburned, wind-burned, or irritated.

This mask acts as a gentle exfoliant. The buttermilk's slight bleaching action can help even out blotchy skin tone if it is used at least twice per week. Mix this recipe as needed; do not store.

1   tablespoon finely ground oatmeal or oat flour

2–3   teaspoons buttermilk

YIELD: 1 treatment

PREP TIME: 5 minutes

TO MAKE

Combine the ground oats and buttermilk in a very small bowl and mix thoroughly with a small whisk or spoon. Let the mixture thicken for a few minutes, then give it a few stirs again to remove any lumps. If it's too thick, add a tad more buttermilk; if it's too thin, add more oats.

TO APPLY

Using your fingers, spread the oat mixture onto your face and throat. Lie down and relax for 20 to 30 minutes. When you're finished, rinse off with warm water.

Use as desired. Follow with moisturizer.

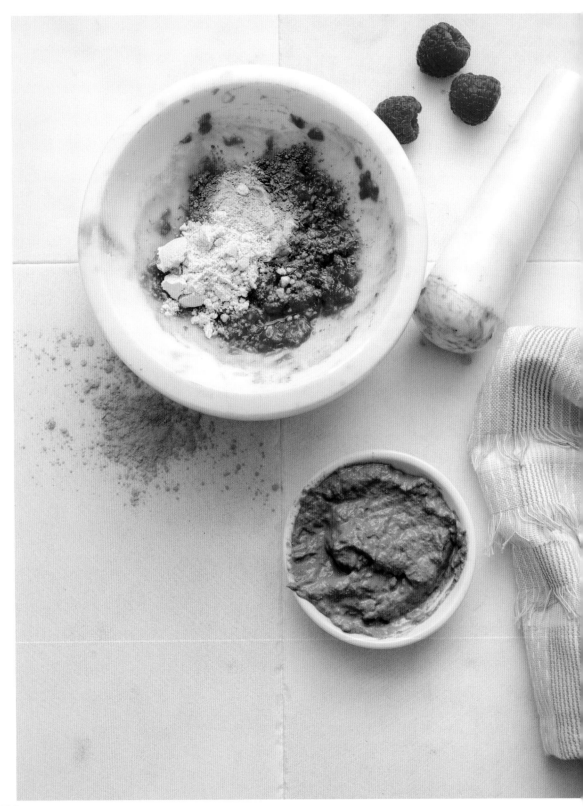

RASPBERRY REFINING MASK

This mask gently exfoliates, tightens, smooths, and brightens dull, slack, blotchy skin, leaving behind a "raspberry" radiance. Mix this recipe as needed; do not store.

1/4 cup raspberries*

1–2 teaspoons purified water (if berries aren't very juicy)

2 teaspoons finely ground oatmeal or oat flour

2 teaspoons powdered white cosmetic or kaolin clay

*Try substituting frozen raspberries for fresh berries; just thaw them ahead of time.

TO MAKE

Using a mortar and pestle or a small bowl and fork, mash the raspberries until nearly smooth. This should produce a runny pulp. Don't worry about the seeds; they should be included. If the berries are on the dry side, add a little water until the pulp is quite juicy. Add the oats and clay and stir until the mixture forms a spreadable paste. Let the mixture sit for a minute or two to thicken. If the mixture seems too thick, add more water; if it's too thin, add more clay or oats.

TO APPLY

Using your fingers, spread the paste onto your face and throat. Lie down with a towel wrapped around your hair and another under your neck. Relax for 20 to 30 minutes. When you're finished, rinse off with warm water.

Use one or two times per week. Follow with moisturizer.

SKIN TYPES RECOMMENDED FOR all, except dry or sensitive

Avoid if your skin is sunburned or windburned; use as tolerated on environmentally damaged skin.

YIELD: 1 treatment

PREP TIME: 10 minutes

RECOMMENDED FOR
puffy, baggy, tired
eyes surrounded by
dehydrated skin

Poof! NO MORE PUFFY EYES MASK

YIELD: 1 treatment

PREP TIME: 35 minutes

This mask hydrates and tightens skin, diminishes puffiness, and leaves eyes feeling refreshed. Mix this recipe as needed; do not store. If you wear contact lenses, remove them before applying this mask.

2 teaspoons peeled, seeded, and finely grated cucumber or raw potato

1 teaspoon plain yogurt

TO MAKE
- - - - - - - - - - - - - - - -

Combine the ingredients in a very small bowl and stir into a smooth, medium-thick paste. Set in the refrigerator to chill for 30 minutes.

TO APPLY
- - - - - - - - - - - - - - - -

Lie down, close your eyes, and apply the mixture to the entire eye area, including the lids. As it warms, the consistency will loosen, so be sure your hair is tucked up out of the way. Relax for 10 minutes, then rinse off with cool water.

Use one or two times per week. Follow with moisturizer.

After using the mask on page 122, try this rinse.

REFRESHING RINSE *for* TIRED EYES

This herbal remedy is very refreshing and soothing to tired, irritated, swollen eye tissue. It feels especially wonderful when the liquid is very cold — it actually perks you up physically and mentally. If you wear contact lenses, remove them before using this rinse.

Note: Because you'll use this product on your eyes, it's especially important that your storage container is sterilized with hot soapy water and bleach or run through the dishwasher prior to storing this rinse.

RECOMMENDED FOR
tired, dry, irritated, or bloodshot eyes

YIELD: 1 cup

PREP TIME: 45 minutes

- 1 cup distilled water
- 1 tablespoon dried eyebright, chamomile flowers, or fennel seeds, or 2 tablespoons fresh

TO MAKE

In a small saucepan, bring the water to a boil and then remove from the heat. If you're using fennel seeds, crush them using a mortar and pestle. Add the herb of your choice to the hot water, cover, and let steep for about 30 minutes. Pour the liquid twice through a strainer lined with cheesecloth, muslin, or a coffee filter to remove all particulate matter. Pour into a storage bottle or spritzer. Label and date.

TO STORE

Refrigerate for up to 7 days, then discard.

TO APPLY

Keeping your eyes open as best you can, splash or mist the infusion over your eyes. You could also use this infusion with an eye cup, which is available at most pharmacies.

Use as desired.

Tips
EYE SOOTHERS

Cold temperatures constrict blood vessels, decreasing puffiness, redness, and irritation. To help relieve puffiness and dark circles, apply any of the following to your eyes, and then lie back and rest for 15 minutes:

- Cold, damp black or green tea bags

- Cosmetic cotton rounds soaked in chilled tea of catnip, rose petals, chamomile flowers, elder flowers, eyebright, fennel seeds, lavender buds, or blackberry leaves

- Thin slices of cold cucumber or white potato

- Cosmetic cotton rounds soaked in cold witch hazel

- Cosmetic cotton rounds soaked in cold, full-fat coconut milk or whole dairy milk

- Chilled rose, chamomile, lavender, or lavandin hydrosol, spritzed directly into and around the eyes or used as an eye wash

You can also try using chilled metal teaspoons. Place four metal teaspoons in ice water to chill. Leave two spoons chilling and take two spoons and apply one to each eye, with the concave side toward your skin, following the contour of the eye socket. When the spoons begin to warm, switch them with the spoons still chilling in the ice water. Continue, alternating spoons, until puffiness subsides or for up to 20 minutes.

Facial Steams

Herbal facial steams have an almost magical ability to transform a dreary, sluggish, parched, lackluster complexion into a dewy, glowing, supple, younger version of itself. Warm, moist heat encourages the pores to perspire and breathe. Steam also imparts vital moisture to deeper skin layers, relaxes muscle tissue, plumps wrinkles, boosts circulation, and brings oxygenated blood to the skin surface. Finally, steam coaxes the facial tissues to relinquish toxins. As the steam penetrates the skin, the various herbs release their volatile oils, which act as astringents or tonics to aid in repair and rejuvenation. Any clogging from sebum, dirt, or makeup is dislodged for easy removal, thus causing pores to appear less visible.

Preparation Tips

If you'd like to make a larger batch of your favorite herbal facial steam mixture to have handy for yourself or gift giving, place the dry ingredients in an airtight ziplock bag, plastic or glass jar, or tin and store it in a dark, cool place, where it will keep for 6 to 12 months. Add the water and oil or vinegar whenever you're ready for a facial steam.

After you've steamed your face, if the leftover herbal liquid doesn't contain vinegar, essential oils, or base oils, let it cool, strain it, and use it to water your plants. If it does contain any of these ingredients, add it to your bathwater or pour the whole mixture onto your compost pile. It needn't go to waste!

CONTRAINDICATIONS

Herbal steams may be used regularly by all skin types with the exception of people who have weepy active or cystic acne; heat-sensitive, sunburned, or windburned skin; or skin with dilated capillaries or rosacea. Heat can further irritate these conditions.

RESTORATIVE HERBAL STEAM

This mixture contains soothing, remedial, and slightly astringent herbs to help balance and tighten all skin types. It can double as a softening, brightening hair rinse for light brown, blond, or red hair. To use as a hair rinse, strain, cool, and pour the entire recipe over your hair after conditioning. Mix this recipe as needed; do not store.

YIELD: 1 treatment

PREP TIME: 15 minutes

3 cups distilled or purified water

2 teaspoons dried blackberry, raspberry, or strawberry leaves or 4 teaspoons fresh, chopped

1 teaspoon dried calendula blossoms or 2 teaspoons fresh, chopped

1 teaspoon dried chamomile flowers or 2 teaspoons fresh

1 teaspoon dried peppermint leaves or 2 teaspoons fresh, chopped

TO MAKE AND USE

Follow the directions for facial steams on page 54.

Use one or two times per week. Follow with moisturizer.

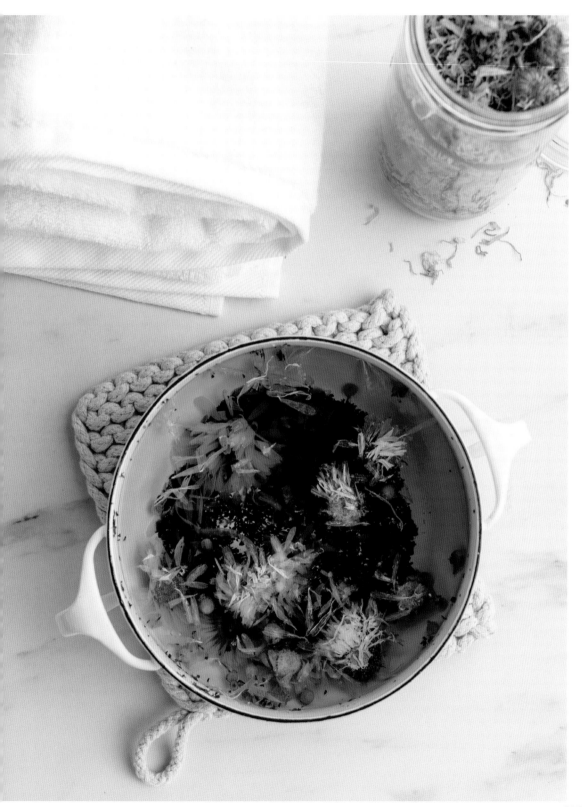

YIELD: 1 treatment

PREP TIME: 15 minutes

SKIN BALANCING STEAM

This facial steam is particularly effective if you wear either pressed or loose powder foundation makeup daily or use soap to cleanse your skin — both can leave behind a drying, alkaline film, resulting in patchy dryness, dull skin, and clogged pores. Your skin is naturally a bit on the acid side with a pH of approximately 5.5 to 6. The vinegar in this steam helps restore your skin's proper pH balance and leaves skin feeling fresh and soft. Mix this recipe as needed; do not store.

3 cups distilled or purified water

¼ cup apple cider vinegar

1 teaspoon dried lavender buds or 2 teaspoons fresh

1 teaspoon dried rosemary leaves or 2 teaspoons fresh, chopped

1 teaspoon dried rose petals or 2 teaspoons fresh, chopped

TO MAKE AND USE

Follow the directions for facial steams on page 54. Please make sure your eyes are closed while taking this steam; the vinegar may sting or cause your eyes to become irritated and water excessively.

Use one or two times per week. Follow with moisturizer.

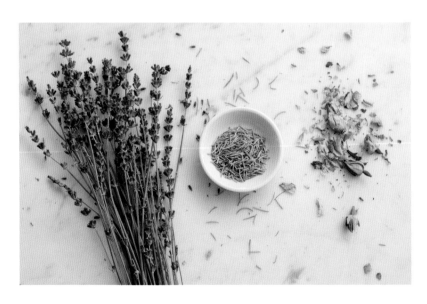

DRY SKIN SAUNA

This steam is like a gentle spring rain for your skin: hydrating, refreshing, and softly stimulating. It's my go-to steam during the winter months when indoor air can further parch my already dry skin. Mix this recipe as needed; do not store.

SKIN TYPES RECOMMENDED FOR
all, except oily or combination

For contraindications see page 125.

YIELD: 1 treatment

PREP TIME: 15 minutes

3 cups distilled or purified water

1 teaspoon dried calendula blossoms or 2 teaspoons fresh, chopped

1 teaspoon dried comfrey leaves or 2 teaspoons fresh, chopped

1 teaspoon dried elder flowers or 2 teaspoons fresh

1 teaspoon favorite base oil

TO MAKE AND USE

Follow the directions for facial steams on page 54.

Use one or two times per week. Follow with moisturizer.

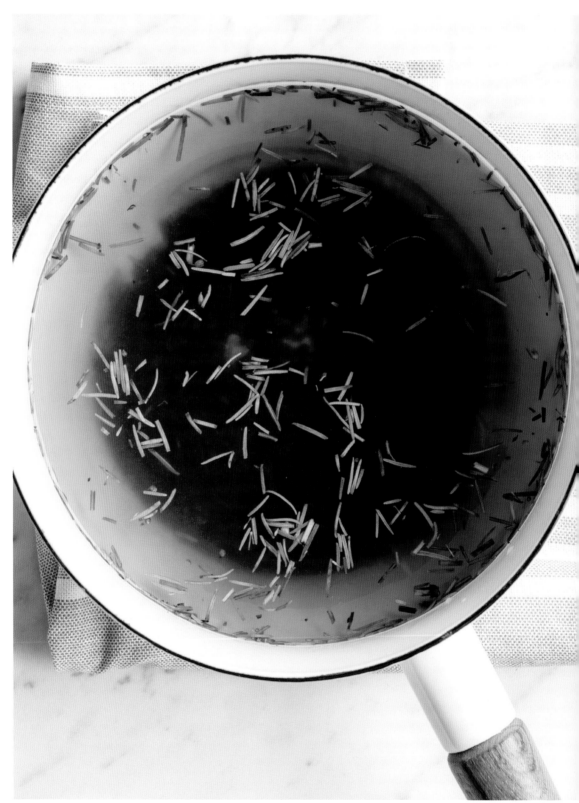

REFRESHING PORE CLEANSER

SKIN TYPES
RECOMMENDED FOR
normal
oily
combination
oily mature

For contraindications see page 125.

All the herbs in this mix have the ability to tighten the skin, combat excessive oiliness, and stimulate circulation. Mix this recipe as needed; do not store.

YIELD: 1 treatment

PREP TIME: 15 minutes

3 cups distilled or purified water

1 teaspoon dried peppermint leaves or 2 teaspoons fresh, chopped

1 teaspoon dried rosemary leaves or 2 teaspoons fresh, chopped

1 teaspoon dried sage leaves or 2 teaspoons fresh, chopped

1 teaspoon dried yarrow flowers or 2 teaspoons fresh, chopped

TO MAKE AND USE

Follow the directions for facial steams on page 54.

Use one or two times per week. Follow with moisturizer.

STRESS-REDUCING EXPRESS STEAM

YIELD: 1 treatment

PREP TIME: 5 minutes

Both lavender and geranium oils can help balance sebum production in the skin and gently improve poor circulation. The aroma of this steam helps reduce stress and anxiety and relieve fatigue. Mix this recipe as needed; do not store.

3 cups distilled or purified water

3 drops geranium essential oil

3 drops lavender essential oil

TO MAKE AND USE

Follow the directions for facial steams on page 54.

Use one or two times per week. Follow with moisturizer.

Good to Know

AROMATHERAPEUTIC EXPRESS FACIAL STEAMS

These two facial steam recipes don't require blending and brewing herbs but simply call for the use of highly therapeutic essential oils — meaning they take less time to prepare than the previous herbal steam recipes. No steeping needed!

Essential oils are concentrated and have varied and multiple properties. When you take these steams, your entire being will reap a wealth of healing goodness.

DELICATE FLOWER EXPRESS STEAM

SKIN TYPES RECOMMENDED FOR
all, except oily or combination

For contraindications see page 125.

This steam is designed especially for delicate, thin, damaged skin lacking in vitality, suppleness, and tone. Mix this recipe as needed; do not store.

YIELD: 1 treatment

PREP TIME: 5 minutes

3   cups distilled or purified water

4   drops neroli or lavender essential oil

2   drops frankincense (CO_2) essential oil

TO MAKE AND USE

Follow directions for facial steams on page 54.

Use one or two times per week. Follow with moisturizer.

Scrubs

As we've learned, the epidermis sheds millions of dead cells daily. The rate at which your body renews its skin slows as you age, however, so gentle exfoliation becomes increasingly important to maintaining healthy, supple skin. If these dead cells remain on your skin, they can form a thick layer of buildup, creating a semi-impenetrable barrier to any moisturizers you apply. This leaves your skin thirsty and prone to wrinkles, and it will rapidly show its age. Manual exfoliation aids the body in its natural shedding process. It also helps loosen ingrown hairs, stimulate circulation, and lift away dirt and excess sebum without the use of drying soap.

Exfoliant facial scrubs are used to remove dry, dead skin cells from the delicate surface of the skin on your face and neck. Unlike many commercial facial scrubs that contain harsh, gritty pumice, ground apricot kernels, walnut hulls, or plastic beads (which are also an environmental no-no), the recipes here contain softer, soothing ingredients that accomplish the same goal while being much easier on the skin.

Many people, especially those who wear minimal or no makeup, may prefer to use a facial scrub instead of a foaming, cream, or lotion cleanser for daily cleaning. The facial scrubs here cleanse, exfoliate, and nourish and never strip protective oils from the skin.

Exfoliant body scrubs give the skin a healthy radiance, help it retain more moisture and flexibility, and keep it youthful-looking longer. I prefer granulated organic brown or white sugar as the primary base for my body scrubs, since it never stings, but it can be physically irritating to sensitive and thin skin unless used with great care. In addition to being an abrasive exfoliant, sugar acts on a chemical level: it contains natural glycolic acid, an ingredient that clarifies skin and loosens the bonds that hold skin cells together, allowing them to slough off easily.

Note: The two body scrub recipes at the end of this chapter are strictly for your body; they are too abrasive for the delicate skin on your face, throat, and chest.

Application Tips

When using any of these exfoliants, especially the more granular ones, do not *scrub* your face and neck. They are not the kitchen sink! Your body may be able to tolerate a bit more friction from body brushes, loofahs, and sugar or salt scrubs, but the more delicate skin tissue on your face and neck will not tolerate such rough handling. Please allow the product to do the work for you and be very gentle, avoiding the eye area at all times.

Even when scrubbing your body, be careful not to abuse and irritate your skin by scrubbing too vigorously. A gentle touch is all that's needed.

It's best to apply facial and body scrubs to freshly cleansed, slightly damp skin, which will help the product glide more gently, with less friction, on the skin. Cleansing your face before exfoliating is especially important if you wear heavy makeup or foundation, if you're dirty or greasy, or if you're just plain sweaty.

CONTRAINDICATIONS

Generally, scrubs can be used on all skin types except for people with acne, dilated capillaries or thread veins, rosacea, sensitive and irritated skin, sunburned or windburned skin, or thin, mature, or elderly skin. Some scrubs, however, are considered relatively nonabrasive and can be used by people with even the most sensitive of skin. So if you suffer from one or more of these challenging skin conditions, take heart: a couple of recipes offered here are very gentle yet effective and can help improve the look and feel of your skin.

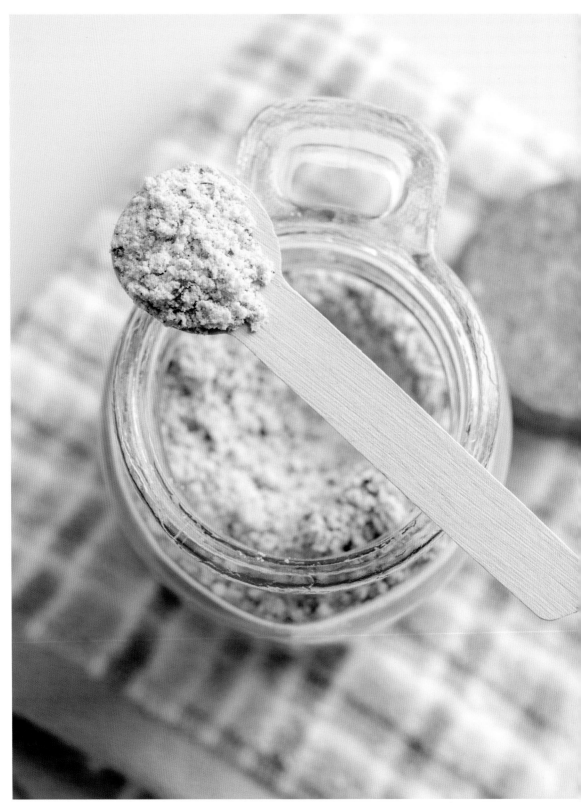

STEPHANIE'S ORIGINAL ALL-PURPOSE SCRUB

SKIN TYPES RECOMMENDED FOR
all

For contraindications see page 135.

YIELD: 1 cup dry ingredients

PREP TIME: 10 minutes

This recipe was the first skin care product I ever made. I was about 15 at the time, and I've used and loved it ever since. It leaves your skin feeling very smooth and doubles as a facial mask: simply apply, let dry for 20 minutes, and then rinse.

1/2 cup ground oatmeal or oat flour

1/4 cup almond meal

1/4 cup sunflower seed meal

1 teaspoon ground, dried peppermint, rosemary, or spearmint leaves

Dash of cinnamon powder (optional, but it adds a pleasant hint of spicy fragrance)

For dry skin: About 2–3 teaspoons full-fat coconut milk, heavy cream, or half-and-half

For normal skin: About 2–3 teaspoons coconut water, almond milk, or low-fat or whole dairy milk

For oily skin: About 2–3 teaspoons distilled or purified water

The liquid quantities given above assume you are using this as a facial scrub. For use as a body scrub, you'll need more liquid. Stir your liquid of choice into the dry mix slowly, adding just enough to make a paste.

TO MAKE

Thoroughly blend all the dry ingredients in a small bowl using a spoon or small whisk, or shake them in a ziplock plastic bag. Pour the mixture into a storage container. Label and date.

TO STORE

No refrigeration is required for the dry scrub mixture, but for maximum freshness and potency, please use within 6 months. Store in a dark, cool cabinet.

Recipe continues on next page

TO APPLY

In a very small bowl, combine 1 tablespoon of the dry scrub mixture (or more if you plan to use it on your body) with enough of the appropriate liquid to form a spreadable paste. Allow the paste to thicken for 1 minute. Using your fingers, gently massage the scrub onto your face and throat for a minute. Rinse well with warm water.

Use daily or as needed. Follow with moisturizer.

Good to Know

WHY EXFOLIATE ON A REGULAR BASIS?

The epidermis, the thin outer layer of the skin that is visible to the eye and protects the body, renews and replaces itself completely every 30 to 60 days or so. This timetable varies with age, health, lifestyle habits, skin care regimen, and environmental factors. The younger you are, the more rapid the cellular turnover and natural sloughing of spent epidermal cells. As you age, the skin's metabolism naturally slows, resulting in slower cell turnover and a buildup of surface dead skin cells. Gentle, consistent exfoliation is essential to aid in the removal of this dry, scaly, lackluster layer, revealing a fresher, smoother complexion that will more readily accept beneficial hydration from a toner, astringent, facial steam, mask, or moisturizer.

OUTTA HERE, OIL! SKIN SCRUB

SKIN TYPES
RECOMMENDED FOR
normal
oily
combination
oily mature

*For contraindications
see page 135.*

Due to the gently astringent witch hazel and sea salt, this scrub is great for oily areas on the shoulders, chest, and back. It doubles as a facial mask: simply apply, let dry for 20 minutes, and then rinse.

YIELD: 1 cup dry ingredients

PREP TIME: 10 minutes

½ cup almond meal	1 teaspoon ground, dried peppermint leaves
½ cup finely ground oatmeal or oat flour	1 teaspoon ground, dried rosemary leaves
1 tablespoon finely ground sea salt	About 2–3 teaspoons witch hazel

The liquid quantity given above assumes you are using this as a facial scrub. For use as a body scrub, you'll need more liquid. Stir the witch hazel into the dry mix slowly, adding just enough to make a paste.

TO MAKE

Thoroughly blend all the dry ingredients in a small bowl using a spoon or small whisk, or shake them in a ziplock plastic bag. Pour the mixture into a storage container. Label and date.

TO STORE

No refrigeration is required for the dry scrub mixture, but for maximum freshness and potency, please use within 6 months. Store in a dark, cool cabinet.

TO APPLY

In a very small bowl, combine 1 tablespoon of the dry scrub mixture (or more if you plan to use it on your body) with enough witch hazel to form a spreadable paste. Allow the paste to thicken for 1 minute. Using your fingers, gently massage the scrub onto your face and throat for a minute. Rinse well with warm water.

Use two times per week. Follow with moisturizer.

MOISTURIZING CREAMY SCRUB

YIELD: 1 treatment

PREP TIME: 5 to
10 minutes

Using this moisturizing scrub frequently will give your skin a "peaches and cream" glow. It doubles as a moisturizing mask: simply apply, relax for 20 minutes, and then rinse. It may be a bit runny, so if you're going to use it as a mask, don a shower cap or wrap your hair in a towel. Mix this recipe as needed; do not store.

¼ small ripe peach, peeled

1 tablespoon full-fat coconut milk or cream (light or heavy)

1 teaspoon dried, powdered chamomile flowers, rose petals, or lavender buds

1 tablespoon finely ground oatmeal or oat flour

1 teaspoon sunflower seed meal

Try doubling the amount of coconut milk or dairy cream and omit the peach if ripe peaches are unavailable.

TO MAKE

Using a mortar and pestle or a small bowl and fork, mash the peach until smooth. Add the rest of the ingredients and blend to form a very creamy paste. If it seems too thin, add more ground oats; if it's too thick, add more liquid. Allow to thicken 1 minute.

TO APPLY

Using your fingers, massage the scrub onto your face, throat, and chest (if desired) for a minute. Then lie down for 5 minutes, leaving the mixture on your skin. Rinse off with warm water.

Use daily or as needed. Follow with moisturizer.

BASIC ALMOND SCRUB

SKIN TYPES RECOMMENDED FOR
all

For contraindications see page 135.

This is a very basic and quickly made scrub. When a larger quantity of the almond meal is blended with your favorite milk and combined with fresh or dried fruit, it makes a delicious nutty snack, too! Mix this recipe as needed; do not store.

YIELD: 1 treatment

PREP TIME: 5 minutes

1 tablespoon almond meal

For dry skin: 2–3 teaspoons full-fat coconut milk, heavy cream, or half-and-half

For normal skin:
2–3 teaspoons coconut water, low fat or whole dairy milk, or vegan milk

For oily skin: 2–3 teaspoons distilled or purified water

TO MAKE

In a very small bowl, combine the almond meal with enough of the appropriate liquid to form a spreadable paste. Allow the mixture to thicken for 1 minute.

TO APPLY

Using your fingers, spread the scrub onto your face and throat and gently massage for a minute. Rinse well with warm water.

Use daily or as needed. Follow with moisturizer.

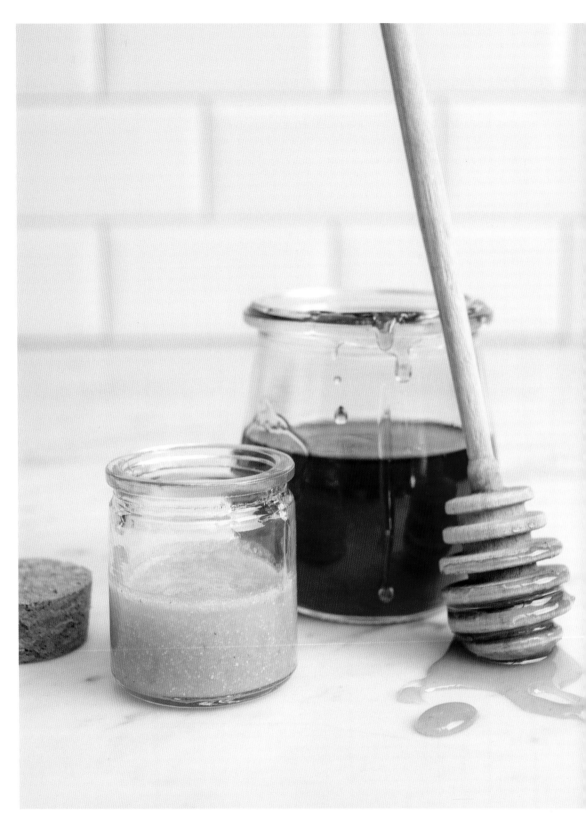

HYDRATING HONEY SCRUB

This product leaves your skin smooth, soft, and very hydrated. Mix this recipe as needed; do not store.

SKIN TYPES RECOMMENDED FOR
all

For contraindications see page 135.

YIELD: 1 treatment

PREP TIME: 5 minutes

1½ teaspoons cornmeal

1 teaspoon raw honey

½ teaspoon distilled or purified water

TO MAKE

In a very small bowl, blend the ingredients thoroughly. Let the mixture sit for 2 to 3 minutes so the cornmeal can absorb the liquids.

TO APPLY

Because this scrub can be a bit runny and sticky, don a shower cap or wrap your hair in a towel before starting. Using your fingers, gently massage the scrub onto your face and throat for a minute. Then lie back for 15 minutes, leaving the scrub on your skin. Rinse well with warm water.

Use two times per week. Follow with moisturizer if needed.

**SKIN TYPES
RECOMMENDED FOR**

normal

dry

mature

environmentally
damaged

*For contraindications
see page 135.*

YIELD: 1 treatment

PREP TIME: 5 minutes

SENSATIONAL SUNFLOWER FRICTION

Apple's malic acid helps this scrub refine the skin's surface by loosening the bonds that bind surface skin cells together, thus stimulating exfoliation of dull, dead skin. This mixture is very hydrating and excellent to use regularly if you live or work in an arid environment. Mix as needed; do not store.

1 tablespoon applesauce

1 tablespoon sunflower seed meal

TO MAKE

In a very small bowl, combine the ingredients to form a spreadable paste. Allow the mixture to thicken for 1 minute.

TO APPLY

This scrub is a bit runny, so don a shower cap or wrap your hair in a towel before starting. Using your fingers, massage the scrub onto your face, throat, and chest (if desired) for a minute. Then lie down for 10 minutes, leaving the scrub on so that the oils of the sunflower seed meal can be absorbed by your thirsty skin. Rinse well with warm water.

Use two or three times per week. Follow with moisturizer.

TROPICAL SKIN-LIGHTENING EXFOLIANT

SKIN TYPES RECOMMENDED FOR
all, except very sensitive

Avoid if your skin is irritated, sunburned, or windburned.

Due to the protein-dissolving enzymes and fruit acids contained in the fresh, raw papaya or pineapple, this treatment, if used repeatedly, will lighten skin discolorations or hyperpigmentation and will generally brighten a lackluster complexion. It's effective to use on sun-damaged, blotchy skin. An ultra-soft, radiantly smooth complexion will be your reward! This exfoliant especially benefits those for whom granular scrubs are contraindicated. Mix this recipe as needed; do not store.

YIELD: 1 treatment

PREP TIME: 5 to 10 minutes

3–4   tablespoons fresh papaya or pineapple (fruit)

TO MAKE

Using a mortar and pestle, mash the fruit until it is smooth and pulpy. Strain the pulp until you have approximately 1 tablespoon of juice.

TO APPLY

Pull your hair up and out of the way prior to application. Saturate a cotton ball or cotton square with the fruit juice and apply to the face, throat, and chest (if desired), until the skin is completely covered by a thin layer of juice. Lie back and allow the juice to dry for 10 to 15 minutes. Rinse with cool water.

Note: It's normal to feel a slight tingle or stinging sensation as the juice dries; this simply means the fruit acids and protein-dissolving enzymes in the juice are doing their job of digesting skin-dulling dead cell debris and brightening your complexion. If the feeling becomes uncomfortable, however, rinse immediately with cool water. Discomfort may indicate that your skin is too sensitive for this treatment.

Use one or two times per week as tolerated. Follow with moisturizer.

SMOOTH-*as*-SILK OATMEAL EXFOLIANT

YIELD: 1 treatment

PREP TIME: 5 minutes

This is a basic multipurpose formula. It can be left on the skin for 20 to 30 minutes to dry as a mask for all skin types; in a larger quantity, it can be used as an effective soap-free daily cleanser for the face or entire body; and it can be used as an extremely gentle scrub. When I travel, I often take with me a ziplock bag with about a cup of oat flour, as it needs no preservatives and won't spoil. What more could you ask from a natural cosmetic? Mix this recipe as needed; do not store.

1   tablespoon oat flour or very finely ground oatmeal

2–3   teaspoons hydrosol of choice or distilled or purified water

TO MAKE

In a small bowl, combine the oats with enough liquid to form a smooth, spreadable paste. Allow the mixture to thicken for a minute. Add more liquid if it's too thick or more oats if it's too thin.

TO APPLY

Using your fingers, massage the mixture onto your face, throat, and chest (if desired) for a minute. Rinse well with warm water.

Use daily if desired. Follow with moisturizer.

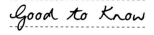

Good to Know

CLOGGED UP?

People sometimes ask me whether scrub ingredients can clog the shower drain. I've never had a problem with this. The salt and sugar dissolve in water within a minute or two of application, and the spices, clay, ground oats, and ground sunflower seeds absorb water and become a slurry that simply rinses off and easily flows down the drain.

HERBAL EXFOLIANT *and* SOAP SUBSTITUTE

SKIN TYPES RECOMMENDED FOR
all

YIELD: 2 cups

PREP TIME: 10 to 15 minutes

I use this formula often when my body skin is dry and I want to avoid soap or a grittier sugar or salt scrub. It thoroughly cleanses without stripping away natural oils, leaving the skin feeling fresh and soft. It doubles as a gentle, soap-free facial cleanser for all skin types and can also be used as a mask: simply apply a thin layer on clean skin, allow it to dry for 20 minutes, then rinse with warm water and pat dry.

- ½ cup powdered dried lavender buds or ¼ cup ground dried orange peel
- ½ cup ground oatmeal or oat flour
- ½ cup sunflower seed meal
- ½ cup powdered white cosmetic clay or kaolin
- 40 drops lavender or sweet orange essential oil (optional)
- About ¼ to ½ cup distilled or purified water or coconut water

TO MAKE

Combine the lavender, ground oats, sunflower seed meal, and white clay in a medium bowl. Blend thoroughly with a spoon or whisk. Add the essential oil, if using, drop by drop and stir or whisk again to completely incorporate. Spoon the mixture into a storage container and seal tightly. Label and date.

TO STORE

No refrigeration is required, but for maximum freshness and fragrance, please use within 6 months. Store in a dark, cool cabinet.

TO APPLY

To mix the scrub for use, scoop ¼ to ½ cup of the dry mixture into a small bowl and add enough liquid to form a spreadable paste. Using your fingers, massage the scrub over your entire body, using circular motions. Rinse well with warm water.

Use daily if desired. Follow with moisturizer.

SWEET *and* SPICY BODY POLISH

YIELD: 2 cups

PREP TIME: 10 minutes

NOTE: This is a body-
only exfoliant; NOT
for use on face.

This is a true sensory delight for the spice lover. The stimulating aroma subtly lingers long after the sugar has been rinsed away, and the scrub provides effective exfoliation with amazing smoothness and lubrication to the skin.

- 1 cup brown sugar
- 1 cup white granulated sugar
- 3/4 cup almond, apricot kernel, jojoba, or sunflower oil

- 2 teaspoons powdered cinnamon
- 2 teaspoons powdered ginger
- 2 teaspoons powdered nutmeg
- 40 drops cardamom essential oil

TO MAKE

Combine all the ingredients except the essential oil in a medium bowl. Blend thoroughly with a spoon or whisk, making sure to break up any lumps of brown sugar or spice. Add the essential oil drop by drop and stir or whisk again to completely incorporate. Spoon the mixture into a storage container and seal tightly. Label and date.

TO STORE

No refrigeration is required, but for maximum freshness and fragrance, please use within 6 months. Store in a dark, cool cabinet.

TO APPLY

Using your fingers, massage 1/4 to 1/2 cup of the scrub over your body, using circular motions. Rinse well with warm water.

Use one or two times per week. Follow with moisturizer if necessary.

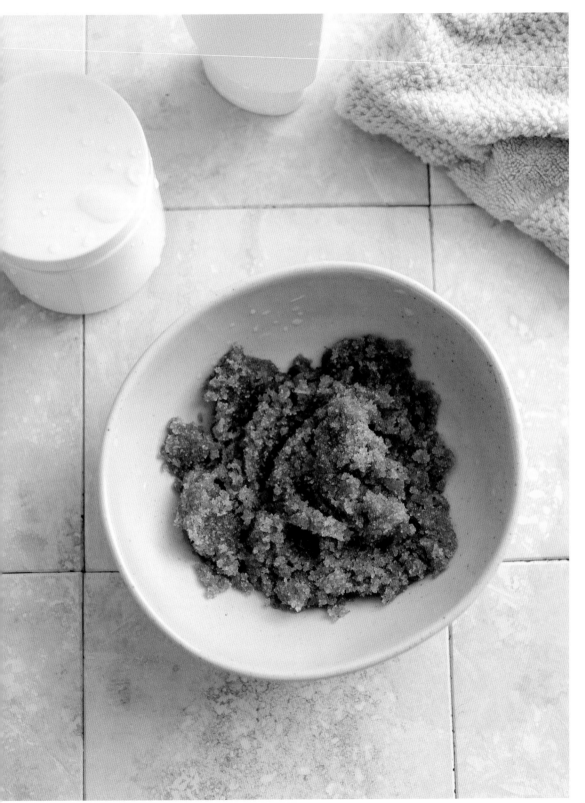

YIELD: 2 cups

PREP TIME: 10 minutes

NOTE: This is a body-only exfoliant; NOT for use on face.

SALT *of the* EARTH BODY SCRUB

This is an ultra-invigorating blend, perfect to use in the morning as a wake-me-up, skin-sparkling scrub. It enlivens all the senses!

2 cups finely ground sea salt

3/4 cup almond, extra-virgin olive, jojoba, or sunflower oil

40–60 drops eucalyptus, grapefruit, peppermint, rosemary (ct. verbenon) or non-chemotype specific, spearmint, or tea tree essential oil

TO MAKE

Combine the sea salt and the almond oil in a medium bowl. Using a spoon or whisk, stir to blend. Add the essential oil drop by drop, and stir again to completely incorporate. Spoon the mixture into a storage container and seal tightly. Label and date.

TO MAKE

No refrigeration is required, but for maximum freshness and fragrance, please use within 6 months. Store in a dark, cool cabinet.

TO APPLY

Using your fingers, massage 1/4 to 1/2 cup of scrub over your body, using circular motions. Rinse well with warm water.

Use one or two times per week. Follow with moisturizer if necessary.

A LITTLE SALTY

Sea salt serves as a remedial agent to the skin when used in moderation, but it can sting and dehydrate irritated, sensitive, sunburned, windburned, thin, fragile, or mature skin. Skin that has just been shaved or waxed will burn when salt is applied; think about walking in the ocean after you've just shaved your legs — ouch! I use a salt scrub when my skin is particularly dirty or I really need to slough rough knees, elbows, palms, and feet. It can be used all over if you are able to tolerate it without discomfort.

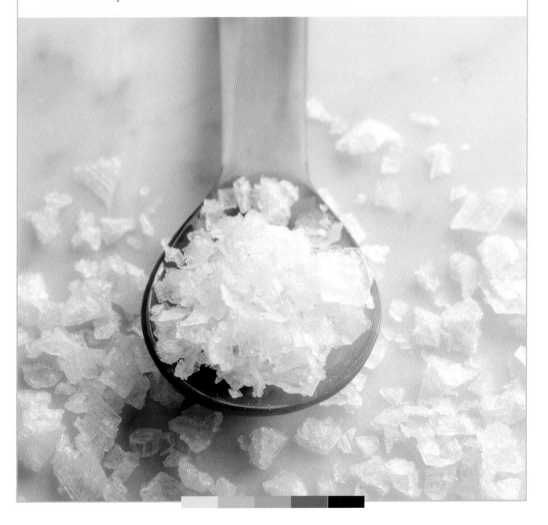

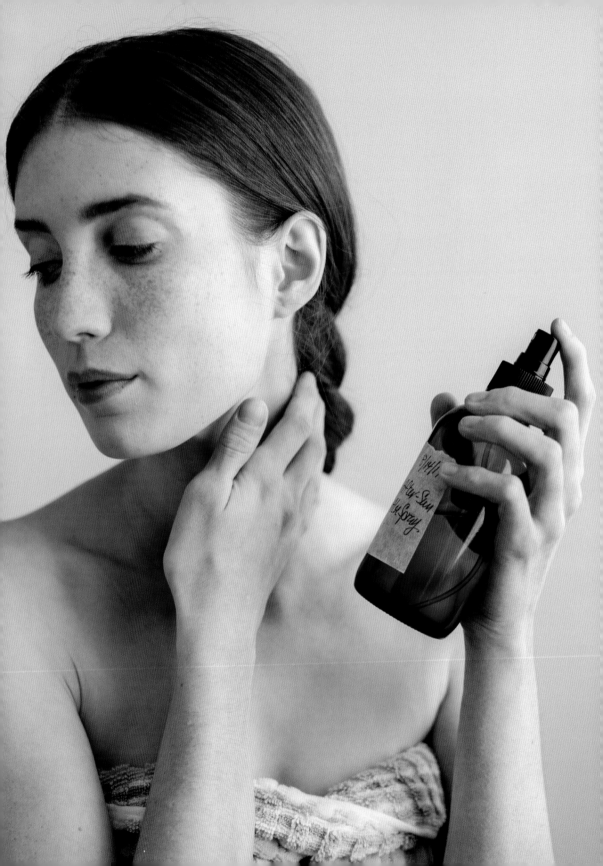

Chapter 6

NOURISH
AND PROTECT

Recipes for Moisturizers,
Elixirs, Skin Conditioners,
and Sun Care

The following recipes will help you take your skin care routine to the next level, ensuring that your largest organ is well-fed, conditioned, lubricated, and shielded from common environmental hazards like dehydrating wind, temperature extremes, and damaging sun, all of which lead to premature aging of the skin. This is crucial no matter what skin type you have, and I recommend many of the recipes in this chapter for use on all skin types. Those with dry or sensitive skin especially will find relief in the formulas that follow.

Facial Moisturizers

Moisturizers can be your skin's best friend. When you apply moisturizer, you are putting a barrier between your skin and a world full of pollutants, dehydrating indoor heat and air-conditioning, and potentially age-accelerating, damaging environmental factors. Moisturizers contain water (or a water-based substance), and they hydrate, soothe, protect, coat, and promote suppleness. Facial oils or elixirs, made from pure base oils and a blend of beneficial essential oils, are not technically moisturizers because they contain no water. They will, however, seal in moisture from the toner, astringent, or hydrosol that you've previously applied to your skin.

Depending upon the skin type for which the moisturizer is created, recipes call for varying quantities and types of water-based and oil-based ingredients. Always use a moisturizer designed for your skin type to avoid overmoisturizing, which makes skin appear oily, or undermoisturizing, which leaves the skin thirsty and dry.

Storage Tips

The moisturizing recipes here contain no preservatives other than vitamin E oil and essential oils, thus they have a relatively short shelf life. They require no refrigeration if used within 60 to 90 days. If your storage area is very warm, please use these natural products within 30 days. If a homemade moisturizing cream is stored in the refrigerator unopened, it may keep for up to 6 months or more. Refrigeration may unfavorably change the product's consistency, but its potency will be preserved.

Application Tips

Unless otherwise specified, apply moisturizers and facial elixirs to freshly cleansed skin following the use of toner, astringent, or hydrosol and immediately following facial treatment such as a scrub, steam, or mask. Don't forget to moisturize or apply a facial oil to your neck and chest twice daily. Many people neglect these areas, which can actually reveal the aging effects of sun exposure and chronological years sooner than your face.

LIGHT and LIVELY MOISTURIZER

Use this very light, hydrating moisturizer anytime your skin needs to be refreshed or is feeling tight and dry. The glycerin acts as a skin-softening humectant, drawing moisture from the air to your skin. This moisturizer is especially beneficial for those with normal, oily, combination, sunburned, or windburned skin.

YIELD: $1/2$ cup

PREP TIME: 5 minutes

- $1/2$ cup distilled or purified water

- 1 teaspoon vegetable glycerin

- 5 drops carrot seed, frankincense (CO_2), geranium, grapefruit, lavender, lemon, or rosemary (ct. verbenon) essential oil

TO MAKE

Combine all the ingredients in a 4-ounce storage bottle or spritzer and shake vigorously to blend. Label and date.

TO STORE

No refrigeration is required, but for maximum freshness and potency, please use within 6 months. Store in a dark, cool cabinet.

TO APPLY

Shake well before use. This product can be applied to your face and throat with a cotton ball or pad or by spraying the skin lightly and allowing to dry. It may even be spritzed lightly over makeup to add dewy freshness.

Use daily.

COCOA BUTTER LOTION

This nongreasy, deeply moisturizing and hydrating rich lotion doubles as a fabulous after-sun skin conditioner. Especially beneficial for those suffering from sunburn or windburn, it leaves skin very soft and silky with a light, velvety orange Creamsicle scent. In summer, I use this as one of my head-to-toe moisturizers.

YIELD: 2 cups

PREP TIME: 30 minutes, plus 30 minutes to set up and cool

1/2 cup unrefined coconut oil

1/4 cup almond, apricot kernel, jojoba, macadamia nut, or sunflower oil

2 tablespoons shea butter (refined or unrefined)

1 tablespoon beeswax or vegetable emulsifying wax

1 tablespoon cocoa butter

1 cup plus 1 tablespoon distilled or purified water

1 teaspoon vegetable glycerin

10 capsules 200 IU vitamin E oil

30 drops sweet orange essential oil

30 drops tangerine essential oil

20 drops vanilla essential oil (CO_2 or absolute)

Try substituting an additional 30 drops of sweet orange essential oil for tangerine essential oil.

TO MAKE

Following the Making Creams and Lotions technique on page 58, heat the coconut oil, almond oil, shea butter, beeswax, and cocoa butter until just melted. In another pan, warm the water and glycerin, stirring gently. Remove both pans from the heat. Pour the oil/butter/wax mixture into a blender and allow it to cool for approximately 20 minutes, or until it begins to turn slightly opaque.

Place the lid on the blender and remove the lid's plastic piece. With the blender turned on medium speed, slowly drizzle the water and glycerin mixture into the vortex of swirling fats below. Almost immediately the cream will turn off-white to very pale yellow and will begin to thicken. Blend for 10 to 15 seconds, or until all the watery mixture has been added, then check the consistency of the cream. It should have a smooth, glossy texture.

Turn off the blender and the add vitamin E oil (pierce the capsule skin and squeeze out the contents) and the essential oils. Blend for another 5 seconds or so, until the cream is smooth and thick.

TO STORE

The lotion will keep best in a dark, cool cabinet. Use within 60 to 90 days. If your storage area is very warm, please use the lotion within 4 weeks for maximum potency and freshness. On the day that you notice any mold growing in your container, toss it out and make a fresh batch.

TO APPLY

Apply $1/2$ to 1 teaspoon over your entire face, throat, and chest, and more as necessary for your body.

Use daily.

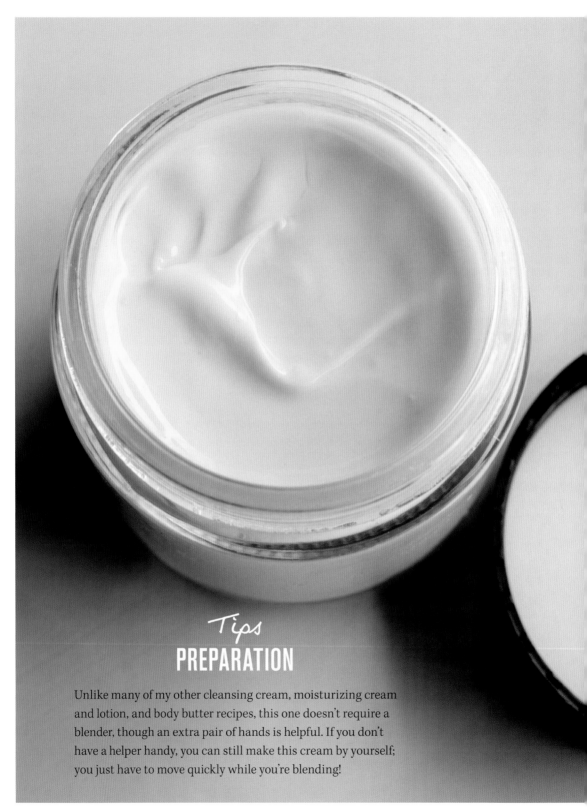

Tips
PREPARATION

Unlike many of my other cleansing cream, moisturizing cream and lotion, and body butter recipes, this one doesn't require a blender, though an extra pair of hands is helpful. If you don't have a helper handy, you can still make this cream by yourself; you just have to move quickly while you're blending!

RICH *and* ROYAL REGENERATING CREAM

SKIN TYPES RECOMMENDED FOR
all, except oily or combination

YIELD: $1/4$ cup

PREP TIME: 30 minutes, plus 1 hour to set and synergize

This is an intensely fragrant, hydrating, skin-plumping, luxurious cream fit for a queen — or king! Though the recipe makes only a small amount, a little goes a long way. The exotically aromatic essential oils and rose hip seed oil are nourishing, act as cellular regenerators, and promote vitality within the skin. The cream is best used in the evening, as the essential oils have gentle tranquilizing properties.

- 1 tablespoon plus 2 teaspoons almond, sunflower, jojoba, or macadamia nut oil

- 2 teaspoons rose hip seed oil

- $1^1/_2$ teaspoons beeswax or vegetable emulsifying wax

- 1 teaspoon shea butter (refined or unrefined)

- 1 tablespoon distilled or purified water or lavandin, lavender, neroli, rose, or rose geranium hydrosol

- $1/4$ teaspoon vegetable glycerin

- 1 capsule 200 IU vitamin E oil

- 10 drops geranium or lavender essential oil

- 10 drops neroli, sweet orange, or lavender essential oil

- 5–10 drops ylang ylang, rose otto, or lavender essential oil

TO MAKE

Heat

In a very small saucepan over low heat or in a double boiler, warm the base oils, beeswax, and shea butter, stirring a few times, until the solids are just melted. In another tiny pan, gently warm the water and vegetable glycerin, and stir a few times until the glycerin dissolves in the liquid.

Recipe continues on next page

Cool

Remove both pans from the heat and let their contents cool almost to body temperature, until the oils/wax/shea butter mixture *just barely* begins to turn opaque but is still liquid. This happens quickly, within 2 to 3 minutes, depending on the temperature of your kitchen, so keep an eye on it.

Blend

Quickly drizzle the watery mixture into the oils/wax/shea butter mixture, stirring rapidly with a small spoon or whisk as you go. Continue stirring rapidly for 2 to 4 minutes, or until a rich gold emulsion forms.

Add the vitamin E oil (pierce the capsule skin and squeeze out the contents) and the essential oils, then rapidly stir for another 4 to 5 minutes, or until the mixture is cool. This recipe really gives your forearm a workout! You should now have a moderately thick, shiny golden cream.

Package and Cool

Spoon the cream into a beautiful storage container — it looks gorgeous in a cobalt-blue glass jar. The product should be cool enough that you can cap the jar immediately so none of the volatile essential oil constituents escape into the air. Label and date the jar. Allow the cream to set and synergize for at least 1 hour prior to use.

TO STORE

The cream will keep best in a dark, cool cabinet. Use within 60 to 90 days. If your storage area is very warm, please use the cream within 4 weeks for maximum potency and freshness. On the day that you notice any mold growing in your container, toss it out and make a fresh batch.

TO APPLY

This cream is highly concentrated; you'll need only a pea-size amount to cover your face and throat and a little more to cover your chest and breasts, if you wish. Rub the cream between your palms to warm it before applying, then massage it into your skin.

Use daily.

SAY GOODNIGHT *to* WRINKLES EYE THERAPY

SKIN TYPES RECOMMENDED FOR
all, except oily

YIELD: 1 treatment

This simple treatment is deeply conditioning and softening and helps keep dry, crinkly wrinkles at bay. I find the light application of oil extremely soothing to the area around my eyes, especially if I've been outdoors in glaring sun (and forgot my sunglasses) or have spent hours staring into a computer screen.

1/4   teaspoon almond, apricot kernel, avocado, extra-virgin olive, jojoba, macadamia, or sesame oil

TO APPLY

Cleanse and tone your face, leaving it slightly damp, especially the eye area. Pour a few drops of your chosen base oil into the palm of your hand — approximately 1/4 teaspoon will do.

Dip your ring finger into the oil and gently pat the substance around (not directly on) your eye in this fashion: Begin at the outer corner and slowly move beneath your eye toward the inner corner, then onto the very upper portion of the lid or brow bone area just below the actual brow, and back over to the outer corner. Do this several times, then pat off any excess oil, leaving a light film of oil on your skin.

Use daily. Follow with moisturizer.

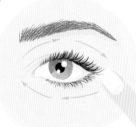

Caution: The reason for not applying the oil directly onto the lid and lashes is that if any of the oil were to get into your eye, it could potentially clog your tear ducts and cause puffiness (which we're trying to avoid!). The delicate eye area acts like a wick and will draw the moisture and lipids (fats) it needs from the surrounding plump, healthy skin tissue.

Herbal Facial Elixirs

When I first heard about the highly touted "youthifying" commercial facial serums that many cosmetics companies were launching in the mid-1990s, I decided to see what all the hoopla was about. These little bottles of promise came at a hefty price, and after a bit of ingredient sleuthing, I discovered that they consisted primarily of water, synthetic skin softeners, chemical exfoliating acids, a vitamin or two, humectants, artificial fragrance, and preservatives. To say the least, most were unsavory cocktails for your face!

So I decided to create my own highly beneficial natural versions of these serums. The result: herbal facial elixirs (also known as facial oils) that your skin will literally drink! If used consistently, the elixirs here will definitely aid in prolonging the youthful qualities of your skin.

Think of the following recipes as alternative moisturizing treatments for your face. Instead of applying a traditionally made cream or lotion, first moisten your skin with your favorite toner, astringent, or hydrosol, then apply one of these specialized blends of pure base and essential oils. They'll nourish on a cellular level, restore, soften, balance, condition, and help repair damaged skin. Expect visible results after regular use. As an added benefit, the aromatherapeutic properties of these elixirs will serve to calm, uplift, recharge, or soothe the mind and spirit.

Preparation and Storage Tips

The prep time for these recipes is minimal, but plan on setting aside your elixir for at least 1 day after making it. Have you ever heard the expression "The sum is greater than its parts"? There's a scientific term for that: *synergy*. During the 24 hours that you let your blend rest, you are letting it synergize, so that it becomes a more powerful conditioner for your skin.

Herbal elixirs do not require refrigeration and should be used within 6 months. If your storage area is very warm, please use within 3 months. Specific storage requirements are included with each recipe.

Application Tips

Unless otherwise specified, herbal elixirs should always be applied to freshly cleansed skin following the use of your favorite toner, astringent, or hydrosol and immediately following any facial treatment such as a scrub, steam, or mask.

Don't forget to apply your conditioning elixir to your neck and chest as well. Many people neglect these areas, which can actually reveal the aging effects of sun exposure and chronological years sooner than your face.

EVENING LUXE ELIXIR

YIELD: 1 ounce

PREP TIME: 15 minutes, plus 24 hours to synergize

This elixir is designed for all skin types in need of light pampering and balancing. It softens, conditions, rejuvenates, aids in healing, tones the skin, and speeds cell regeneration. The base oils penetrate and should leave no oily residue. Combined, the essential oils have a calming, sedative effect on the psyche and body. Applying this just before bedtime can help lull you into restorative sleep.

8 drops neroli essential oil

4 drops frankincense essential oil (CO_2)

4 drops lavender essential oil

4 drops rose otto essential oil

1 tablespoon hazelnut oil

1 tablespoon jojoba oil

TO MAKE

Add the essential oils, drop by drop, directly into a glass storage bottle. Add the base oils. Screw on the dropper bottle top, wrap your hand around the bottle, and shake the formula vigorously for 2 minutes to completely blend all the ingredients and gently warm them to body temperature. Label and date. Set the bottle in a dark location that's between 60°F (16°C) and 70°F (21°C) for 24 hours so that the oils can synergize.

TO STORE

No refrigeration is required, but for maximum freshness and potency, please use within 6 months. Store in a dark, cool cabinet.

TO APPLY

Immediately before bedtime, cleanse your face, then apply the appropriate toner, astringent, or hydrosol. While your skin is still damp, place 10 to 15 drops of the elixir into the palm of one of your hands, rub both palms together, and then lightly massage the elixir into your skin, beginning with your chest and throat and then moving to your face, using upward, outward, and circular strokes. Wait 5 minutes before applying additional moisturizer (if desired).

Use one time per day, right before bedtime.

OUT, DAMN SPOT! ANTIBLEMISH ELIXIR

SKIN TYPES RECOMMENDED FOR
any with active blemishes

This elixir, with broad-spectrum antiseptic properties, is specifically designed to zap subsurface acneic bacteria, ridding skin of irritating toxins and associated redness. It's excellent to use on infected ingrown hairs that can form after a bikini wax, bikini-line shave, or the shaving of tough beard hair. This product is also great for soothing itchy bug bites.

YIELD: ½ ounce

PREP TIME: 15 minutes, plus 24 hours to synergize

- 4 drops tea tree essential oil
- 2 drops clove essential oil
- 2 drops German chamomile essential oil
- 2 drops green myrtle essential oil
- 2 teaspoons hazelnut or apricot kernel oil
- 1 teaspoon almond oil

TO MAKE

Add the essential oils, drop by drop, directly into a glass storage bottle. Add the base oils. Screw on the dropper bottle top, wrap your hand around the bottle, and shake the formula vigorously for 2 minutes to completely blend all the ingredients and gently warm them to body temperature. Label and date. Set the bottle in a dark location that's between 60°F (16°C) and 70°F (21°C) for 24 hours so that the oils can synergize.

TO STORE

No refrigeration is required, but for maximum freshness and potency, please use within 6 months. Store in a dark, cool cabinet.

TO APPLY

Before applying, cleanse the blemished area with your regular cleanser, astringent, toner, or hydrosol. Then place 1 or 2 drops of elixir into the palm of your hand, dip a cotton swab into the oil, and dab onto each pimple.

To use on infected ingrown hairs: Apply 1 drop to each area displaying irritation and/or infection and massage in with your fingertips.

Use one or two times per day.

HEALING THYME ELIXIR

YIELD: 1 ounce

PREP TIME: 15 minutes, plus 24 hours to synergize

This elixir helps balance problem skin due to overactive sebaceous glands. The combination of essential oils produces a formula with antibacterial properties that also calms the skin, counteracting redness from inflammation. It also aids in normalizing dry areas, improves sluggish circulation, and stimulates new cell formation.

8 drops German chamomile essential oil

5 drops rosemary (ct. verbenon) essential oil

5 drops thyme (ct. linalool) essential oil

2 drops lemon essential oil

2 tablespoons hazelnut oil

TO MAKE

Add the essential oils, drop by drop, directly into a glass storage bottle. Add the base oil. Screw on the dropper bottle top, wrap your hand around the bottle, and shake the formula vigorously for 2 minutes to completely blend all the ingredients and gently warm them to body temperature. Label and date. Set the bottle in a dark location that's between 60° (16°C) and 70°F (21°C) for 24 hours so that the oils can synergize.

TO STORE

No refrigeration is required, but for maximum freshness and potency, please use within 6 months. Store in a dark, cool cabinet.

TO APPLY

Every morning and evening, after cleansing, apply the appropriate toner, astringent, or hydrosol. While your skin is still damp, place 10 to 15 drops of the elixir into the palm of one of your hands, rub both palms together, and then lightly massage the elixir into your skin, beginning with your chest and throat and then moving to your face, using upward, outward, and circular strokes. Wait 5 minutes before applying sunscreen, additional moisturizer, or makeup.

Use two times per day.

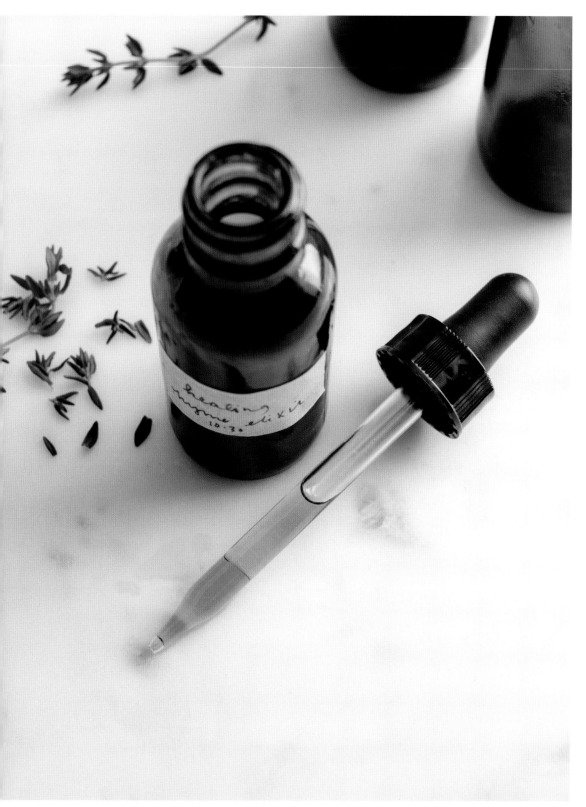

REPAIR and RESTORE REMEDY

YIELD: 1 ounce

PREP TIME:
15 minutes, plus
24 hours to synergize

This is a regenerative elixir containing anti-inflammatory properties and skin-supportive fatty acids that help repair and pamper environmentally stressed and mature skin, leaving behind a healthy feel, more even tone, and suppleness. It can be especially beneficial for those with sunburned or windburned skin. This blend can also be used to help prevent stretch marks, to speed post-operative skin rejuvenation, and to aid in healing mild first-degree burns.

- 7 drops carrot seed essential oil
- 7 drops helichrysum essential oil
- 6 drops calendula essential oil (CO_2)

- 1 tablespoon apricot kernel oil
- 1 teaspoon macadamia nut oil
- 1 teaspoon rose hip seed oil
- 1 teaspoon tamanu oil

TO MAKE

Add the essential oils, drop by drop, directly into a glass storage bottle. Add the base oils. Screw on the dropper bottle top, wrap your hand around the bottle, and shake the formula vigorously for 2 minutes to completely blend all the ingredients and gently warm them to body temperature. Label and date. Set the bottle in a dark location that's between 60°F (16°C) and 70°F (21°C) for 24 hours so that the oils can synergize.

TO STORE

No refrigeration is required, but for maximum freshness and potency, please use within 6 months. Store in a dark, cool cabinet.

TO APPLY

Every morning and evening, after cleansing, apply the appropriate toner, astringent, or hydrosol. While your skin is still damp, place 10 to 15 drops of elixir into the palm of one of your hands, rub both palms together, and then lightly massage the elixir into your skin, beginning with your chest and throat and then moving to your face, using upward, outward, and circular strokes. Wait 5 minutes before applying sunscreen, additional moisturizer, or makeup.

Use two times per day (or three times per day to soothe minor burns or sunburn).

To help prevent scar tissue formation and speed skin repair: To new injuries with the potential for scar formation, apply this elixir by the drop twice daily until the injury is healed. *Please consult with your health care provider prior to usage, especially if you want to use this formula on recent surgical incisions.* To help fade scar tissue that already exists, apply this elixir by the drop twice daily directly to scars anywhere on the body. Scars that are less than 2 years old will tend to respond more favorably than older scar tissue.

To aid the healing of burns: You can use this elixir to help mend mild burns that don't require a physician's care, including sunburns, grease burns, and general "kitchen accident" burns. Immediately pour chilled aloe vera juice onto the area to stop inflammation and cool the tissue. Pat dry. Follow this with an application of several drops of this elixir (or more depending on the size of the burn). Repeat this procedure up to three times per day. You should see dramatic improvement and recovery.

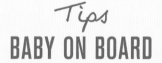

Tips
BABY ON BOARD

To help prevent stretch marks on a pregnant belly, combine ½ to 1 teaspoon of rose hip seed oil with 1 drop of calendula essential oil (CO_2), or 1 drop of lavender essential oil if calendula is unavailable. Apply directly to your expanding abdomen and massage the oil into the entire area. Repeat twice daily. *These are very safe oils,* but check with your health care provider first if you are concerned.

Body Oils, Butters, and Balms

All-natural skin conditioners, whether rich and heavy or light and silky, improve the skin's barrier function by sealing in moisture and preventing evaporation. They also lubricate your skin, improving overall suppleness and elasticity. Applying some type of nurturing conditioner, be it a hydrating moisturizer, silky body oil, or thick butter or balm, is a daily essential, a vitally important skin care step that should never be skipped.

Application Tips

To most effectively seal in your skin's moisture and keep out dehydrating air, apply these products immediately following a bath or shower, after you've toweled off, but while your skin is still slightly damp.

Because body oils, butters, and balms are thick, heavy, rich emollients, a little goes a long way. Begin by using a small amount, like 1 teaspoon, and see how far it spreads. Really massage it into your skin. Apply more or less product depending on the size of the application area; you be the judge. If after 5 minutes your skin has an oily residue, you've used too much. Simply wipe the excess with a towel and use less next time.

BUTTERY BODY OIL

SKIN TYPES RECOMMENDED FOR
all, except oily and combination

In addition to being one of the best all-over skin softeners, this blend is excellent as a spot treatment for dry heels, knees, and elbows and makes a perfect nightly cuticle conditioning oil. With its warm, softly spicy, stimulating scent, this oil is recommended for those who don't enjoy overly floral fragrances.

YIELD: ½ cup

PREP TIME: 20 minutes, plus 24 hours to completely thicken

- 6 tablespoons sesame oil
- 2 tablespoons shea butter (refined or unrefined)
- 2 capsules 200 IU vitamin E oil
- 10 drops cardamom essential oil
- 10 drops ginger essential oil
- 10 drops sweet orange essential oil

TO MAKE

In a small saucepan over low heat or in a double boiler, warm the sesame oil and shea butter until the shea butter is just melted. Remove from the heat and gently stir for 1 minute to blend the ingredients, then allow the mixture to cool to body temperature. Add the vitamin E oil (pierce the capsule skin and squeeze the contents into the mix) and essential oils and stir again. Pour into storage container(s) — plastic squeeze bottles work perfectly — and cap, label, and date.

Note: Because shea butter takes a long time to fully thicken, this formula will need about 24 hours to completely set up. When it's ready, it will be thick and a pale creamy-yellow color. If you've used unrefined shea, your balm will be a hint darker. Unrefined shea butter has a strong scent that will greatly diminish the aroma of the essential oils but not their beneficial properties.

TO STORE

No refrigeration is required, but for maximum freshness and potency, please use within 6 to 12 months. Store in a dark, cool cabinet.

TO APPLY

Immediately following a bath or shower, while your skin is still damp, slather this oil blend on your body — really massage it in. Because it's very concentrated, begin with 1 teaspoon at a time.

Use daily or as desired.

LAVENDER PROTECTION BALM

In the cooler months, I often slather this balm all over my body right before bedtime, especially on areas that need extra attention, such as rough shins, knees, hands, and feet. The soothing, relaxing aroma — a delectable blend of cocoa butter and lavender — is subtle, warm, and soft.

¼ cup almond, jojoba, or sunflower oil

3 tablespoons unrefined coconut oil

1 tablespoon beeswax or vegetable emulsifying wax

2 teaspoons cocoa butter

2 capsules 200 IU vitamin E oil

48 drops lavender essential oil

TO MAKE

In a small saucepan over low heat or in a double boiler, warm the almond oil, coconut oil, beeswax, and cocoa butter until the solids are just melted. Remove from the heat and allow the mixture to cool for 5 to 10 minutes. Add the vitamin E oil (pierce the capsule skin and squeeze the contents into the mix) and essential oil, then gently stir with a small spoon for about 1 minute to blend. Pour the balm into storage container(s) and cap, label, and date. Let it set overnight to give the cocoa butter plenty of time to completely harden.

Note: If the room temperature is above 76°F (24°C), the balm will maintain a softer consistency. If the temperature is below 76°F, the balm will be firmer.

TO STORE

No refrigeration is required, but for maximum freshness and potency, please use within 1 year. Store in a dark, cool cabinet.

TO APPLY

Immediately following a bath or shower, while your skin is still slightly damp, slather your body with this balm. Because it's very concentrated, begin with 1 teaspoon at a time. If your skin has an oily residue after 5 minutes, you've used too much. Simply wipe off the excess with a coarse towel. You can also use the balm as a spot treatment on extra-dry areas of your body.

Use daily or as desired.

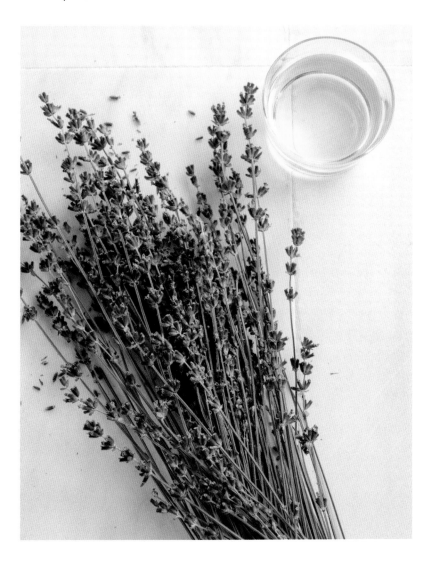

BABY'S BOTTOM BALM

I originally created this balm for infants and small children to protect against diaper rash and soothe occasional bouts of dermatitis, but I've discovered that it also makes a great "ski balm" or barrier balm for times when your skin is going to be exposed to cold, dry air or cold, windy weather. It also makes a great treatment for ragged cuticles and conditions cracked heels, elbows, and rough knees or other dry or rashy skin.

YIELD: ¼ cup

PREP TIME: 20 minutes, plus 12 hours to completely set

2 tablespoons almond, sunflower, extra-virgin olive, or jojoba oil

1 tablespoon cocoa butter

1 tablespoon shea butter (refined or unrefined)

1 teaspoon beeswax or vegetable emulsifying wax

1 capsule 200 IU vitamin E oil

2–4 drops Roman chamomile, lavender, or sweet orange essential oil

TO MAKE

In a small saucepan over low heat or in a double boiler, warm the almond oil, cocoa butter, shea butter, and beeswax until the solids are just melted. Remove from the heat and gently stir with a small spoon for about 1 minute, then allow the mixture to cool for about 5 minutes. Add the vitamin E oil (pierce the capsule skin and squeeze out the contents) and essential oil and stir again to thoroughly blend. Pour into storage container(s) and cap, label, and date. Allow it to set overnight to give the cocoa and shea butters plenty of time to completely harden.

Note: If you've used unrefined shea, your balm will be a hint darker. Be aware that unrefined shea butter has a strong scent that will greatly diminish the aroma of the essential oils but not their beneficial properties.

TO STORE

No refrigeration is required, but for maximum freshness and potency, please use within 1 year. Store in a dark, cool cabinet.

TO APPLY

A little goes a long way, so be judicious with the quantity you apply. This balm can be applied wherever your skin is dry or moisture needs to be sealed in and dehydrating air sealed out. The balm performs best when applied over slightly damp skin.

Use as desired.

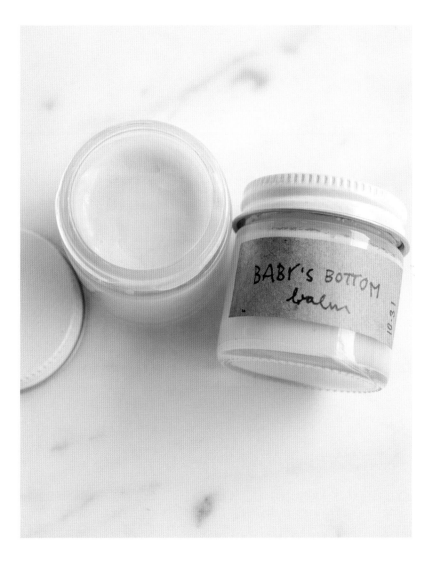

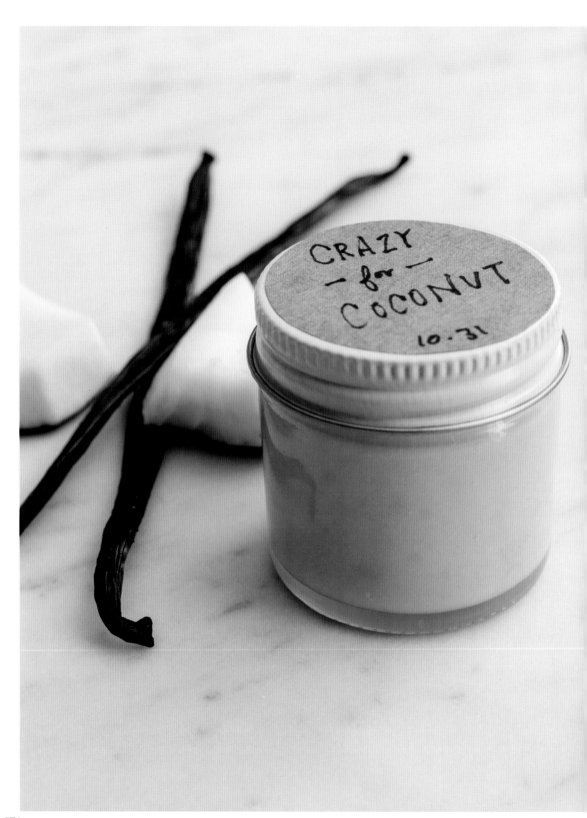

CRAZY *for* COCONUT BALM

SKIN TYPES RECOMMENDED FOR
all, except oily and combination

This product smells luscious, tastes delicious (it's safe to taste — with or without adding the essential oils), and is simple to make. Many people swear by coconut oil's ability to melt right into the skin and use it from head to toe year-round as a superb body beautifier.

YIELD: ½ cup

PREP TIME: 20 minutes, plus 12 to 24 hours to thicken

- 7 tablespoons unrefined coconut oil
- 1 tablespoon cocoa butter
- 2 capsules 200 IU vitamin E oil

- 16 drops peppermint, spearmint, sweet orange, or vanilla (CO_2 or absolute) essential oil (optional)

TO MAKE

In a small saucepan over low heat or in a double boiler, warm the coconut oil and cocoa butter until the butter is just melted. Remove from the heat and let cool for 15 minutes. Add the vitamin E oil (pierce the capsule skin and squeeze out the contents) and essential oil (if desired) and stir to blend. Pour into storage container(s) and cap, label, and date. Allow the mixture to set for 12 to 24 hours to thicken completely.

Note: If the temperature of your storage area is above 76°F (24°C), the balm will maintain a liquid consistency. If the temperature is below 76°F, the balm will be firm. Remember, too, that coconut oil and cocoa butter will melt on contact with skin.

TO STORE

No refrigeration is required, but for maximum freshness and potency, please use within 1 year. Store in a dark, cool cabinet.

TO APPLY

Immediately following a bath or shower, while your skin is still damp, slather this oil blend on your body — really massage it in. A little goes a long way, so begin with 1 teaspoon at a time.

Use daily or as desired.

CHAMOMILE and OLIVE BODY BUTTER

YIELD: 2¼ cups

PREP TIME: 30 minutes, plus 30 minutes to completely cool and set

This herbal butter deeply feeds your skin from the outside and especially benefits inflamed, irritated skin. It also makes a fabulous cleansing cream and facial moisturizer for all skin types and a wonderful nail conditioning cream. It even works well as an antifrizz hair conditioner if applied sparingly to the ends of dry, fine, frizzy hair, and it is a great anti-inflammatory after-sun cream. If you want to use the chamomile-infused oil in lieu of plain extra-virgin olive oil, either make your own (see Oil of Sunshine on page 182 for instructions) or purchase chamomile-infused oil from better health-food stores, a local herb shop, or mail-order herb suppliers.

¾ cup extra-virgin olive oil or chamomile-infused olive oil

¼ cup unrefined coconut oil

2 tablespoons beeswax or vegetable emulsifying wax

1 tablespoon shea butter (refined or unrefined)

1 cup distilled or purified water or chamomile, lavandin, lavender, or rosemary hydrosol

1 teaspoon vegetable glycerin

10 capsules 200 IU vitamin E oil

30 drops German chamomile essential oil

30 drops Roman chamomile essential oil

TO MAKE

Heat

In a small saucepan over low heat or in a double boiler, warm the olive oil, coconut oil, beeswax, and shea butter until the solids are just melted. In another small pan, warm the water or hydrosol and the vegetable glycerin, and stir a few times until the glycerin dissolves in the liquid.

Recipe continues on next page

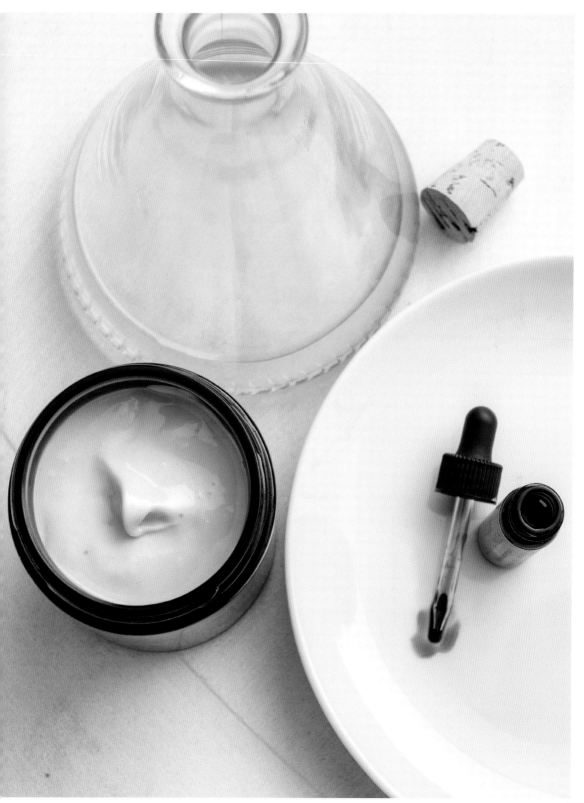

Cool

Remove both pans from the heat. Pour the oils/wax/shea butter mixture into a blender and allow it to cool for approximately 5 to 10 minutes, or until it begins to turn slightly opaque. The time will vary depending on the temperature of your kitchen.

Do not walk away and forget what you're doing and allow this mixture to get too thick or it will not blend properly and you may have a difficult time getting it out of your blender.

Blend

Place the lid on the blender and remove the lid's plastic piece. Turn the blender on medium speed. Slowly drizzle the water and glycerin through the center of the lid into the vortex of swirling fats below. Almost immediately the cream will turn off-white to very pale yellow and will begin to thicken.

If the watery mixture is not properly combining with the fatty mixture, turn off the blender and give the body butter a few stirs with a spatula, being sure to scrape down any residue from the sides of the blender container. Then replace the lid and blend on medium speed for another 5 to 10 seconds. Repeat this process once or twice more, if necessary, until the texture is smooth.

Turn off the blender and add the vitamin E oil (pierce the capsule skin and squeeze the contents into the mix) and essential oils. Put the lid back on, then blend for another 5 seconds or so, until the body butter is smooth and thick. It should be a pale greenish-blue color.

Package and Cool

Spoon the finished body butter into storage container(s). Lightly cover each container with a paper towel and allow the blend to cool for about 30 minutes before capping and labeling.

TO STORE

This body butter is best stored in a dark, cool cabinet. Use within 60 to 90 days. If your storage area is very warm, please use the butter within 4 weeks for maximum potency and freshness. On the day that you notice any mold growing in your container, toss it out and make a fresh batch.

If, after a few hours or days, water begins to separate from your body butter, don't worry. You can pour off the watery liquid and use the resulting super-thick product as a foot, shin, knee, or elbow balm. The mixture can separate if the temperature of the fatty ingredients and that of the watery ingredients are not relatively equal and cool enough when the two portions are blended. Keep trying — making perfect creams and butters is an art!

TO APPLY

Immediately following a bath or shower, slather this butter on your damp skin — really massage it in. Because it's very concentrated, begin with 1 teaspoon at a time. If your skin has an oily residue after 5 minutes, you've used too much. Simply wipe off the excess with a towel and use less the next time around.

Use daily.

Try making your own
infused oil to use
with the body butter
recipe on page 178.

YIELD: 3 to 3½ cups

PREP TIME: 15 minutes,
plus 1 month to infuse

OIL *of* SUNSHINE

This calming oil makes a wonderful conditioning oil for your face
or body and a bath oil for all skin types except oily, acneic, and
combination skin. It's also perfect for infants with diaper rash and can
be used to help heal minor skin irritations, to relieve muscle pain, and
to soothe a young, active child before bedtime. It's one of my favorites!

You'll need a 1-quart sterilized canning jar for this recipe. To sterilize
it, boil it for 10 minutes and then let it thoroughly air-dry.

3 parts dried chamomile
   flowers

1 part dried lavender buds

3-4 cups extra-virgin olive oil

4 capsules 1,000 IU vitamin E
   oil (or 20 capsules 200 IU
   vitamin E oil)

25 drops lavender essential oil

15 drops German chamomile
    essential oil

15 drops Roman chamomile
    essential oil

TO MAKE

Fill the Jar

Loosely fill a dry, sterilized 1-quart canning jar with the chamomile and lavender flowers. They should reach to within an inch or so of the top of the jar.

Drizzle the olive oil over the flowers until the oil comes to within 1 inch
of the top of the jar. The flowers will settle with the weight of the oil, so
don't worry if it looks as though you don't have enough flowers in the
jar. Make sure all plant matter is submerged and none is exposed to air.
The jar should be quite full; there shouldn't be more than 1 inch of space
between the contents and the lid. Add more oil if necessary. Gently stir
with a clean knife or chopstick to remove any trapped air bubbles.

Infuse

Place a piece of plastic wrap or small plastic bag over the mouth of the jar (to avoid having the metal jar lid come into contact with the herbs) and tightly screw on the lid. Shake the jar several times to blend the herbs and oil thoroughly.

Place the jar in a warm, sunny location such as a south-facing windowsill or — if daytime temperatures are consistently above 75°F (23.8°C) — outside on your deck and allow the flowers to solar-infuse for 1 month. Shake the jar for 30 seconds or so daily.

Filter and Blend

After 1 month, carefully pour the oil through a strainer lined with a fine filter such as muslin or, preferably, a paper coffee filter, then strain again if necessary to remove all herb debris. Squeeze the flowers to extract all of the oil. Next, add the vitamin E oil (pierce the capsule skin and squeeze out the contents) and essential oils and stir well to blend.

Note: If mold forms in your jar during the month of infusion, discard the product and begin again, being sure that your jar is sterilized and thoroughly dry.

Pour the finished oil into storage containers (a funnel comes in handy for this).

TO STORE

No refrigeration is required if the oil is used within 6 months. For longer storage of up to 1 year, refrigerate the oil.

Tanning Potions and After-Sun Relief

In chapter 1, I addressed the health benefits of sun exposure and the importance of appropriate sun protection to prevent potential skin damage, but it's important to reiterate that if you want to preserve the beauty and integrity of your skin for years to come and help prevent skin cancer, you *must not* spend excessive unprotected time in the sun. As with all things in life, the sun should always be taken in moderation.

Practice holistic sun care:

Avoid chemical sunscreens, but do find a natural one that works and offers full-spectrum protection.

Use common sun sense by staying out of the sun or wearing appropriate cover-up clothing during the high-intensity hours between 10 A.M. and 2 P.M.

After sun exposure, always slather on a good-quality moisturizing lotion or cream, from head to toe, to prevent further epidermal dehydration.

The natural sun protection recipes that follow have an SPF of approximately 10 or lower and are formulated to nourish and condition your skin before, during, and after exposure to the sun and associated elements such as heat, drying wind, salt water, and chlorine from pools. I've also tossed in a few suggestions for natural remedial action when sunburn does occur.

SUN-SOOTHING BODY OIL

SKIN TYPES RECOMMENDED FOR
all, except oily or acneic, or combination

The ingredients of this recipe combine to form a very hydrating, skin-nourishing blend that helps protect skin from the elements. But should you find yourself suffering from sunburn, windburn, or an itchy rash from sea, sand, salt, or chlorine after a day in the sun, this formula is ultra-soothing and aids in healing the irritation.

YIELD: 1 cup

PREP TIME: 15 minutes

- 1/4 cup commercial aloe vera juice
- 1/4 cup unrefined coconut oil
- 1/4 cup jojoba oil
- 1/4 cup sesame oil
- 5 capsules 200 IU vitamin E oil

TO MAKE

Combine all the ingredients (pierce the vitamin E oil capsules and squeeze the contents into the mix) in an 8-ounce storage container; a plastic squeeze bottle is perfect. Label and date.

TO STORE

No refrigeration is required if the product will be used within 3 weeks or so. If refrigerated, the blend will keep for 4 to 6 months. It will thicken when chilled but will liquefy when warmed to room temperature.

TO APPLY

The aloe vera juice, being water-based, will separate from the oils during storage, so shake well before use. Apply to your entire body immediately before and repeatedly during sun exposure. It's also wonderful to use as an after-sun skin conditioner, especially if your skin is irritated from environmental assaults. Massage the blend into your skin thoroughly. If your skin has an oily residue after 5 minutes, you've used too much. Simply wipe off the excess with a coarse towel.

Use before, during, and after sun exposure.

TROPICAL TANNING BODY OIL

This oil is designed for the die-hard sun worshipper who tans easily and rarely burns. Its SPF is low but its aroma is oh-so-sweet! It may make you want to bake in the sun all day — but don't! Even those who tan easily experience skin damage from excessive sun exposure. This oil is highly emollient and beneficial for any part of the body in need of softening.

YIELD: 1 cup

PREP TIME: 20 minutes,
plus 12 hours to thicken

$1/2$ cup unrefined coconut oil

$1/2$ cup jojoba oil

5 capsules 200 IU
vitamin E oil

1 tablespoon cocoa butter

A few drops of coconut
fragrance or flavoring oil
(optional)*

*The coconut fragrance or flavoring oil is optional but divinely aromatic. Follow the manufacturer's instructions for the appropriate number of drops for 1 cup of oil.

TO MAKE

In a small saucepan over low heat or in a double boiler, warm the coconut oil, jojoba oil, and cocoa butter until the solids have just melted. Remove from the heat, add the vitamin E oil (pierce the capsule skin and squeeze the contents into the mix), and stir the mixture with a spoon for about a minute to thoroughly blend. Add the fragrance or flavoring oil (if desired) and stir again.

Pour the blend into an 8-ounce storage container — a plastic squeeze bottle is great — and cap, label, and date. Allow the mixture to thicken for 12 hours before use.

Note: If the temperature of your storage area is above 76°F (24°C), the product will maintain a liquid consistency. If it's below 76°F, it will be firmer. To soften before use, set the container in a shallow pan of hot water for 10 to 20 minutes.

TO STORE

Store in a dark, cool cabinet. No refrigeration is required, but for maximum freshness and potency, please use within 2 years.

TO APPLY

Shake well before use. Apply this oil immediately after a bath or shower to seal in moisture and prevent evaporation before heading into the sun. A little goes a long way, so begin with 1 teaspoon. Also apply it during and after sun exposure.

Use before, during, and after sun exposure.

Good to Know

A NOTE ABOUT SUNSCREENS

The aim of a good sunscreen is to prevent the sun's UVA "photoaging" rays and UVB "burning" rays from being able to damage your skin and diminish its natural health and youthful radiance. I believe that the best nontoxic sunscreens on the market today are those that are mineral based, containing minerals such as micronized titanium dioxide or zinc oxide, which act as physical reflective barriers to the sun (as opposed to sunscreens with potentially toxic chemicals that actually absorb and disperse the sun's rays). Most mineral-based sunscreens can be used even by people with sensitive skin, and they are relatively sweat-proof.

AFTER-SUN ALOE SPRAY

This blend, with hydrating and anti-inflammatory properties, soothes and rejuvenates skin damaged by sunburn and windburn. It doubles as a remedial anti-itch spray for those suffering from all manner of skin irritation and bug bites.

YIELD: 1 cup

PREP TIME: 5 minutes

1 cup commercial aloe vera juice

20 drops lavender essential oil

12 drops rosemary (ct. verbenon) essential oil

TO MAKE

Combine all the ingredients in an 8-ounce spray bottle and shake well to blend. Label and date.

TO STORE

Please keep refrigerated and use within 4 to 6 months.

TO APPLY

Shake vigorously before each use. Spray on skin as often as necessary. Keep out of eyes.

Use as necessary.

Tips
SUNBURN RELIEF

- Add 2 cups apple cider vinegar to cool bathwater and soak for 10 to 20 minutes.

- Apply cold aloe vera gel or juice directly to sunburn as often as needed to ease pain and rehydrate damaged tissue.

- Apply cold, strong black pekoe or green tea directly to sunburn with soft, soaked cotton flannel or pads. Repeat as needed.

- Spray chilled lavender, rose geranium, lemon balm, or chamomile hydrosol directly onto sunburned areas to help relieve inflammation.

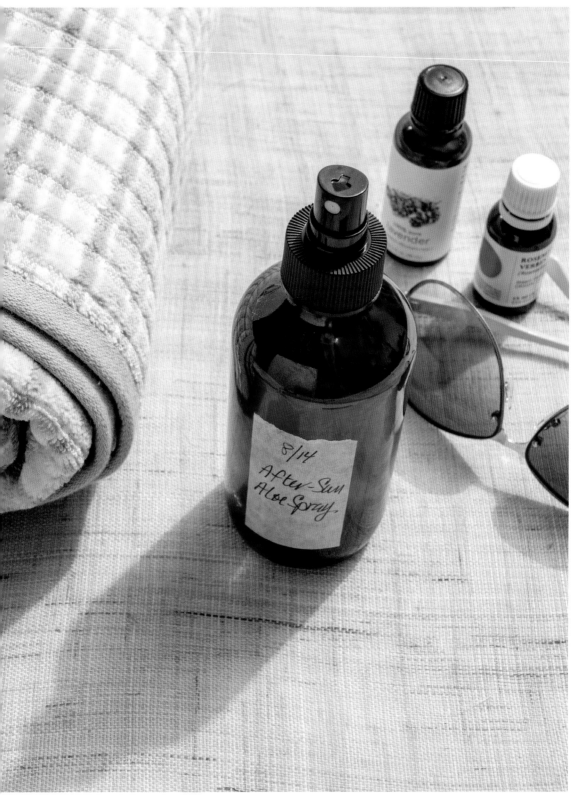

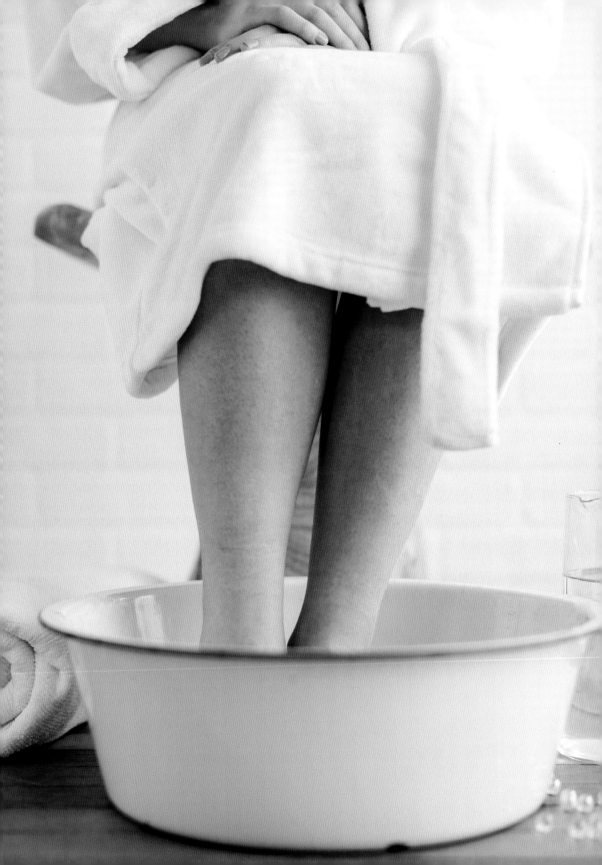

Chapter 7

PAMPER

Recipes for Feet and Hands

The skin on your face is most noticeable to the world, but taking good care of the skin on your feet and hands is vital to your well-being. Plus, doesn't everyone want their feet and hands to look good and feel great, no matter what their age? The recipes in this chapter will help you keep them moisturized, attractive, and healthy.

Foot Care:
Feelin' Footloose
and Fancy-Free

Your feet were designed to be strong, flexible, and durable. Though some people think feet are a beautiful part of the body, most of us would rather hide our tootsies than show them off!

As an esthetician and reflexologist, I have heard many complaints from clients regarding their feet: "They constantly hurt." "My calluses are so thick I have to cut them with a knife." "My toenails are getting narrow, thick, and ugly." "I'm constantly battling foot odor and sweaty feet." Most of these problems are easily rectified.

Ill-fitting footwear can cause myriad foot problems, and you may find that purchasing proper-fitting, "sensible" shoes will solve problems of corns, calluses, chronic aches, and tiredness. Today you can find many shoe styles created with both comfort and fashion in mind. Foot odor, a common and embarrassing problem, can usually be remedied by wearing natural fiber or moisture-wicking socks and shoes that breathe or going barefoot as much as possible. If you have other foot problems, such as bunions, hammertoes, fallen arches or flat feet, excessive perspiration and odor, or toenail fungus that won't go away, see a podiatrist.

For basic care and preventive maintenance, treat your feet with the following recipes, which are designed to bring relief to your tired, rough, itchy, dry, thickened, abused, neglected, and odoriferous dogs.

INVIGORATING FOOT SCRUB

This scrub is quick and easy to make and leaves feet feeling soft, smooth, tingly, and refreshed. Mix this recipe as needed; do not store.

YIELD: 1 treatment

PREP TIME: 5 minutes

¼ cup cornmeal

¼ cup ground oatmeal

1 tablespoon sea salt or table salt

About ⅓ cup purified or tap water

3–4 drops lemon or peppermint essential oil

TO MAKE

Combine the cornmeal, oatmeal, and salt in a small bowl with enough water to form a creamy, gritty paste. If it's too thin, add more cornmeal; if too thick, add more water. Allow to thicken for a minute or so. Add a few drops of the essential oil and stir again.

TO APPLY

Sit on the edge of the bathtub or on a bench in the shower and massage your feet with this mixture — really scrub all those rough areas and between your toes. Rinse and dry thoroughly, and follow with an application of a thick moisturizing cream or balm combined with a few drops of either essential oil.

Use daily or as needed.

Note: Make sure to clean the bathtub right after this procedure, as the large amount of ground meals may continue to thicken and potentially clog the drain.

SOOTHING FOOT SOAK

This recipe softens leathery feet, deodorizes, and helps relieve the itchiness of athlete's foot. Following this foot soak, use a pumice stone or pedicure wand to buff away any softened calluses. Mix this recipe as needed; do not store.

YIELD: 1 treatment

PREP TIME: 5 minutes

2 cups apple cider vinegar

2 tablespoons vegetable glycerin

TO MAKE

Combine the vinegar and glycerin in a foot tub (such as a plastic dishpan) with enough water, warm or cold, to cover your feet and ankles. Swish with your feet to blend.

TO APPLY

Soak your feet for 15 to 20 minutes. Pat dry and follow with a coating of moisturizer or balm.

Use daily or as desired.

Tips
SWEET RELIEF FOR YOUR FEET

Foot rollers are available in health food stores, online, and in shops that sell bath products. They are wonderful for relieving sore, tired feet. I prefer the wooden ones that have raised ridges from one end to the other.

And remember: a foot massage is a luxury to receive! Massage your loved one's clean feet with any base oil mixed with a few drops of your favorite essential oil; peppermint, lavender, sweet orange, cardamom, or ginger are always nice. This is a great way to spend the evening with your "sole" mate!

NO MORE CALLUSES FOOT SOAK

If you use this treatment on a consistent basis, your feet will become softer and healthier, and unsightly calluses will be a problem of the past (provided you're also wearing proper-fitting shoes). You might just decide you want to show off those tootsies! Mix this recipe as needed; do not store.

You'll need a pumice stone or pedicure wand for the scrub part of this treatment.

YIELD: 1 treatment

PREP TIME: 5 minutes

¹⁄₂ cup baking soda ¹⁄₂ cup sea salt or table salt

TO MAKE

Fill a foot tub (such as a plastic dishpan) with enough comfortably warm or hot water to cover your feet and ankles. Add the baking soda and salt and swish with your feet to dissolve them.

TO APPLY

Soak your feet for 15 or 20 minutes, or longer if you have very thick calluses. Remove one foot from the water and, while still wet, gently scrub any calluses with a pumice stone or pedicure wand. When loose skin begins building up on the scrubbing tool, dip it and your foot back into the foot tub, rinse, and begin again if necessary. Repeat the process with your other foot.

When you're done, roughly rub your feet dry and apply a thick cream or your favorite balm, then don natural-fiber socks. This final application will continue to soften your feet throughout the day or overnight.

You can also follow this scrubbing procedure while taking a bath, after your feet have become soft.

Use daily or as needed.

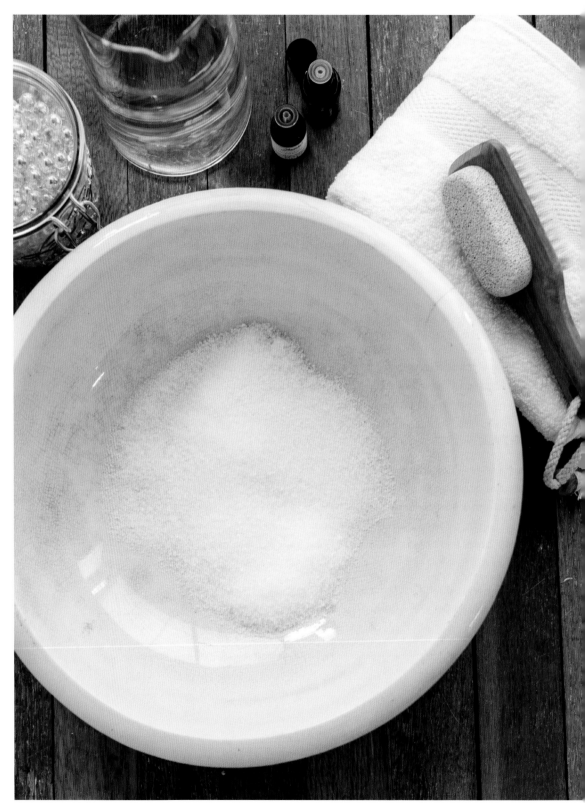

ALL YOUR MARBLES FOOT REFRESHER

RECOMMENDED FOR
tired, achy, swollen feet

The foot exercise and muscle stimulation combined with invigorating essential oils and Epsom salt refresh and relieve achy, swollen feet. This soak is recommended for joggers, walkers, and anyone who is on their feet all day. Mix this recipe as needed; do not store.

YIELD: 1 treatment

PREP TIME: 10 minutes

½ cup Epsom salt

5–10 drops eucalyptus, juniper, lemon, peppermint, rosemary (ct. verbenon or non-chemotype-specific), or sweet orange essential oil

2–3 cups medium marbles

TO MAKE

Combine the Epsom salt and essential oil in a foot tub (such as a plastic dishpan) with enough comfortably hot or cold-as-you-can-stand water to cover your feet and ankles. Swish with your feet to blend, then add enough marbles to almost cover the bottom of the tub.

TO APPLY

Soak your feet for 15 to 20 minutes while gently rolling them back and forth over the marbles. Occasionally grasp and release the marbles with your toes. This action stretches and relaxes the ligaments, tendons, and muscles in your feet. When you're finished soaking, roughly rub your feet dry and apply a soothing lotion mixed with a few drops of one of the essential oils.

Use daily or as desired.

FEELIN' FRESH FOOT POWDER

This recipe makes a very effective deodorizing foot and underarm powder. It can also be used to prevent diaper rash on baby bottoms — but omit the essential oil in this case, please.

YIELD: 2¼ cups

PREP TIME: 15 minutes, plus 3 days for the fragrance to synergize

- 1 cup baking soda
- 1 cup cornstarch
- 2 tablespoons powdered white clay
- 2 tablespoons zinc oxide powder
- 100 drops eucalyptus, lemongrass, peppermint, rosemary (ct. verbenon or non-chemotype specific), sweet orange, tea tree, or thyme (ct. linalool) essential oil

TO MAKE

Combine the baking soda, cornstarch, clay, and zinc oxide in a medium bowl and gently mix with a whisk, or place the ingredients in a food processor and pulse a few times. Add the essential oil a few drops at a time and blend with the whisk, or continue pulsing the food processor as you add the drops.

Transfer the powder to an airtight container and store in a dark, cool place for 3 days to allow the essential oil's fragrance and deodorizing properties to permeate the mixture. After 3 days, package the blend in small shaker containers. Label and date.

TO STORE

No refrigeration is required, but for maximum fragrance and potency, please use within 1 year. Store in a dark, cool cabinet.

TO APPLY

Sprinkle the powder into your shoes and socks once or twice daily, or simply sprinkle onto dry, bare feet whenever desired.

Use daily or as needed.

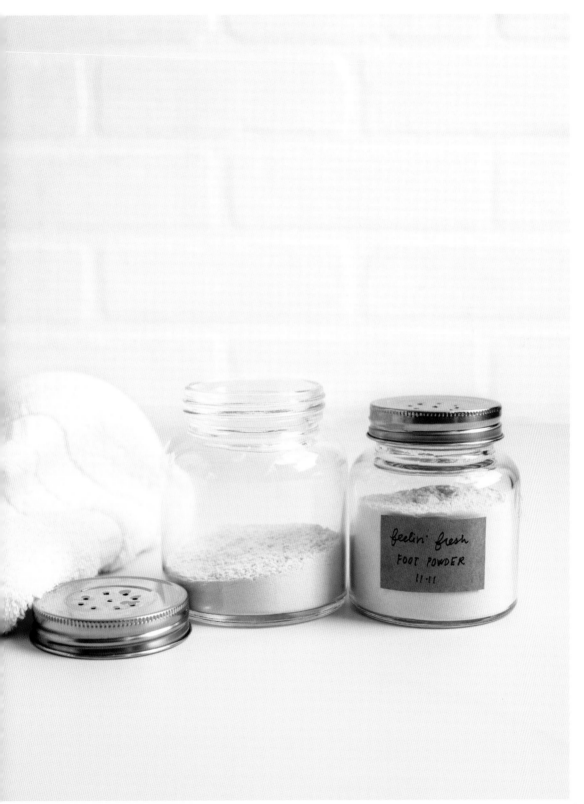

Hand and Nail Treatments

Can you tell what kind of work people do just by looking at their hands? A mechanic's hands and nails will be tough and frequently grease-stained. An office worker's may be smooth and soft, with well-groomed nails. A full-time mother with several children and a small garden will probably have hands sporting short nails and dry skin and cuticles. A carpenter, mason, or farmer may have rough, cracked, suntanned hands with hard fingernails and thick calluses.

We tend to pay a lot of attention to our face and hair but often neglect one of our most expressive features: our hands. They are constantly exposed to sun, wind, heat, cold, harsh cleansers, dirt, and grease and are one of the first places on our body to show age.

You can fight the ravages of time and the elements on your hands by remembering to take a few important steps each day: Apply moisturizer *frequently*; wear appropriate gloves when your hands will be exposed to water, cleansers, or chemicals; and wear garden gloves when you're working outdoors. Don't forget to apply to your hands a natural sunscreen lotion with an SPF of 15 whenever you're in the sun. The following recipes will help to soften, protect, and condition your hands and nails.

RENEWING HAND *and* NAIL BUTTER

No matter which essential oils you choose, this formula is rich, deeply conditioning, and incredibly beneficial for dry, rough, chapped hands and cuticles, chapped lips, and rough knees, elbows, and feet. It's also particularly effective for the prevention of scar tissue when consistently applied to fresh cuts and scrapes.

RECOMMENDED FOR
everyone

YIELD: $1/2$ cup

PREP TIME: 20 minutes, plus 12 hours to completely set

1/4 cup almond, extra-virgin olive, jojoba, or sunflower oil

2 tablespoons cocoa butter

1 tablespoon beeswax or vegetable emulsifying wax

1 tablespoon shea butter (refined or unrefined)

2 capsules 200 IU vitamin E oil

48 drops carrot seed, frankincense (CO_2), geranium, helichrysum, lavender, myrrh, or rosemary (ct. verbenon) essential oil (or any combination)

TO MAKE

In a small saucepan over low heat or in a double boiler, warm the almond oil, cocoa butter, beeswax, and shea butter until the solids are just melted. Remove from the heat and gently stir for 1 minute; then allow to cool for about 5 minutes. Add the vitamin E oil (pierce the capsule skin and squeeze the contents into the mix) and essential oil(s) and stir to blend. Pour into storage container(s) and cap, label, and date.

Note: Cocoa and shea butters take a while to completely set up, so leave the product at room temperature for 12 hours before use. The finished formula will have a paste-wax consistency. Be aware that unrefined shea butter has a strong scent and will greatly diminish the aroma of the essential oil(s) but not their beneficial properties.

Recipe continues on next page

TO STORE

No refrigeration is required, but for maximum freshness and potency, please use within 1 year. Store in a dark, cool cabinet.

TO APPLY

Ideally, apply this blend onto slightly damp hands and feet as an overnight softening treatment, but it can also be applied to dry skin. Wear gloves or socks to seal in moisture and protect sheets.

Use daily or as desired.

For a nail and cuticle treatment: Soak your fingertips in a bowl of warm water for 5 minutes to soften your nails and cuticles. Pat dry. Apply a tiny dab of this butter onto the base of each nail and massage in. Using a small piece of cotton flannel, gently push back your cuticles, and then lightly buff your nails with the cloth. This treatment leaves your fingertips soft and smooth.

For shiny nails: Apply the butter as described above for the nail and cuticle treatment, but use a nail buffer instead of the cloth to gently polish your nails to a soft sheen.

NAIL-STRENGTHENING SOAK

Thick, conditioning castor oil leaves behind a tough, shiny, protective residue on nails, helping to prevent environmental damage. It also strengthens nails and relieves drying and cracking of cuticles.

YIELD: 4 treatments

PREP TIME: 5 minutes

4   tablespoons castor oil

12   drops frankincense (CO_2) or myrrh essential oil

TO MAKE

Combine the castor oil and essential oil in a small bowl — just large enough to comfortably soak your fingertips — and mix with a spoon. Cover the bowl tightly. Label and date.

TO STORE

Refrigerate for up to 1 month, then discard.

TO APPLY

Set the bowl of oil in a shallow hot-water bath for a few minutes until it is comfortably warm. Soak your fingertips in the oil for 5 to 10 minutes to soften your nails and cuticles, then wipe off most of the oil. Using a small piece of cotton flannel, gently push back your cuticles, and then lightly buff your nails with the cloth. You can use the same batch of oil for four soaks.

Use daily or as desired. Follow with moisturizer or balm.

SMOOTH and SOFT HAND PACK

If you use this recipe consistently twice per week, the coloration and texture of the skin on your hands should take on a more uniform appearance. You'll see gradual fading of age spots and hyperpigmentation and should experience enhanced softness and smoothness. This formula, when applied to the face, offers the same benefits, plus it makes pores appear more refined. It's great for all skin types, except very sensitive skin. Simply pull up your hair, place a towel around your shoulders to protect your clothing, and apply the mixture to your face and neck in the same manner as you would to your hands; relax and recline for 20 to 30 minutes, then rinse. Mix this recipe as needed; do not store.

2 tablespoons finely ground oatmeal or oat flour

1 tablespoon fresh lemon juice or fresh, raw apple, pineapple, or strawberry pulp

1 tablespoon plain yogurt

TO MAKE

Combine all the ingredients in a small bowl and stir until the mixture forms a spreadable paste. Allow it to thicken for a minute or so. If the paste is too thick, add a bit of water to thin it slightly; if it's too thin, add more ground oats.

TO APPLY

Apply the mixture to the backs of your hands and allow it to remain for 20 to 30 minutes. Rinse with cool water. Pat almost dry and apply a good moisturizer, balm, or sunscreen.

Use two times per week.

DISINFECTING HAND
and NAIL OIL

RECOMMENDED FOR
minor cuts and scrapes
or for extremely dry,
fissured, rough hands,
knuckles, and cuticles

I like to keep a bottle of this spicy infused oil in the kitchen so that I can use it as a quick first-aid remedy whenever I happen to cut myself while chopping, slicing, or grating. The cloves add mild analgesic and antiseptic properties. This oil also eliminates common kitchen hand odors such as garlic and onion.

YIELD: $1/4$ cup

PREP TIME: 5 minutes, plus 1 month for infusion

- $1/4$ cup almond, extra-virgin olive, jojoba, or sunflower oil
- 1 capsule 200 IU vitamin E oil
- 40 whole cloves

TO MAKE

In a small jar with a tight-fitting lid (a baby food jar is perfect), mix the almond oil, vitamin E oil (pierce the capsule skin and squeeze the contents into the mix), and the cloves. Screw on the lid and place the jar in a warm sunny window for 1 month to allow the cloves to impart their remedial properties to the oil. Shake the mixture daily. The oil will take on a slight amber color, depending on the type of base oil you chose.

At the end of the infusion period, strain out the cloves. Pour the oil into a storage container, label, and date.

TO STORE

No refrigeration is required, but for maximum freshness and potency, please use within 6 months. Store in a dark, cool cabinet.

TO APPLY

Simply apply 1 or 2 drops of the oil to minor skin injuries of the hands and nails or massage a small amount into damp hands as a moisturizing treatment.

Use daily or as needed. Follow with moisturizer if desired.

Appendix

SKIN CARE APOTHECARY

The following pages detail the ingredients called for in the recipes that begin in part two. For your convenience, I list substitutes, when applicable, that you can use when an ingredient called for in a particular recipe is unavailable.

Your local health food store, food co-op, or whole foods grocer is the first place to check for beeswax, cocoa and shea butters, quality essential oils, base oils, raw seeds and nuts, organic herbs, and grains. If you have no luck in your local markets, the Internet, of course, is a go-to resource for just about everything you'll need to create all the recipes in this book. I purchase from mail-order catalogs or Internet sources that I know and trust. I prefer sources that I know have a relatively rapid turnover of stock, so I can be sure the ingredients I purchase are fresh. For a listing of tried and trusted ingredient suppliers, see Resources (page 237).

If you have a green thumb and live in an appropriate climate, you can grow many of the herbs from seed or from herb plants available at your local garden center. Doing so is always a fun and educational project.

Sometimes, while traveling, I get lucky and stumble across a small organic farm that can provide the herbs and oats I use in so many of my skin care formulas. At farmers' markets and local shops, I look for fresh raw honey and beeswax direct from the apiary. Whether you're driving around the countryside, browsing at the market, or just meandering about, keep an eye out for purveyors of farm specialties that you could use in personal care recipes. A fresh ingredient is a first-rate ingredient!

AN INGREDIENT PRIMER

Many of the ingredients listed in the Ingredient Dictionary (page 215) will be quite familiar to you, such as baking soda, sea salt, papaya, honey, and lemon, and my brief description of each one will be sufficient for your complete understanding of its use in personal care recipes. There are four broad categories of personal care ingredients, however, that require a more in-depth introduction: base oils, essential oils, herbs, and meal blends made from seeds, nuts, and oats. In the next few pages you'll come to understand the specific terminology, quality, storage requirements, and preparation techniques for the ingredients in each of these categories. Before you purchase any ingredients and start blending, grinding, mixing, and melting, take a few minutes and educate yourself. Remember: a knowledgeable consumer makes the wisest choices and the highest-quality body care products.

Base Oils

Base oils, also known as carrier oils, are chemically classified as fats — they contain fatty acids and glycerin — and are derived from seeds, nuts, beans, vegetables, flowers, grains, and fruits. Base oils are characteristically greasy, slippery, smooth in texture, and lighter than water, with an extremely low evaporation rate. And, as their name implies, they are used as a base to which we add essential oils, solid fats, thickeners, watery liquids, and herbs and spices to make herb-infused oils, lotions, salves, balms, herbal elixirs, and creams. Base oils can be used alone or in combination with other base oils to create massage oils, bath oils, or makeup-removing products. I use only pure plant-derived oils — never lard, lanolin, cod liver oil, or mineral oil — as I find plant oils to be completely biocompatible with the skin, triggering very few skin sensitivities and having no objectionable odors.

The best base oils for personal care recipes are those that have been naturally extracted and minimally processed from organically grown raw ingredients. The key words to look for on the label are *unrefined*, *expeller-pressed*, or *cold-pressed*. These oils have not been exposed to the extremely high temperatures, chemical extraction procedures, bleaching, or deodorizing that can destroy or alter natural aromas, flavors, antioxidant properties, beneficial vitamins, and trace minerals. These gently processed oils are produced by mechanically pressing the chosen plant matter, then straining out any resulting debris. Some heat is naturally generated during the pressing, but it's not so high that it destroys the vital nutrients, taste, and aroma of the oil. As compared to their highly processed refined cousins, unrefined oils are slightly darker in color, deeper in aroma, truer to taste (if eaten), and much higher in essential fatty acids. They may also have a cloudy appearance at times.

Note that due to superior freshness and lack of processing, unrefined base oils — with the exception of jojoba, extra-virgin olive, and coconut oils — have a short shelf life and tend to become rancid if stored at room temperature for more than 6 to 8 months, especially in warm weather. These oils should thus be refrigerated and used within 1 year. If the oil you are using has a strong or "off" smell (with the exception of extra-virgin olive, tamanu, sesame, or coconut oils; these have naturally strong fragrances), then it's probably old and rancid. Purchase base oils through reputable retailers with a high turnover of inventory. Always check the expiration date on the bottle and never hesitate to return the oil if it's bad.

SLIP AND SLIDE

At times, the terms *slip* and *slide* are used to describe the way an oil or oil-based product glides onto the skin. A particular oil that has a nice slip or slide flows onto the skin effortlessly under mild hand pressure — that is, the oil or product is neither sticky nor too rapidly absorbed. An oil with these properties is perfect to use as a body oil or in balms, butters, lotions, and creams. Organic almond, apricot kernel, coconut, macadamia, and sunflower oils have a thinner texture and excellent slip and slide. Personally, I love extra-virgin olive oil, especially organic Tuscan, for the velvety, slightly heavier texture it imparts to creams, and sesame oil is always a go-to for me because I adore the rich scent. I also like jojoba oil, an excellent balancing body oil, because it's chemically similar to human sebum, leaving desert-dry skin velvety soft and aiding in normalizing oily skin. All three have excellent slip and slide.

Essential Oils

Essential oils are primarily extracted by steam distillation, with the exception of citrus oils, which are cold-pressed from the rind. A newer method of extraction, called supercritical carbon dioxide (CO_2) extraction, is a more expensive process than distillation, but the method yields a higher volume of essential oil. Carbon dioxide also extracts a wider range of molecules than does steam for a more complete and absolutely superior essential oil. It is most often used for the more expensive and/or oil-stingy plant materials, such as frankincense, myrrh, nutmeg, ginger, calendula blossom, and vanilla bean. In this book, when a recipe calls for frankincense or calendula essential oils, I recommend the CO_2 extractions instead of the steam distillations. If the CO_2 version is unavailable, steam-distilled is an acceptable substitute for frankincense but not for calendula, as that steam distilled version smells horrible and can be quite sticky.

Another method used to extract essential oils is solvent extraction, and the resulting oils are referred to as absolutes. Jasmine, rose, hyacinth, vanilla, and mimosa are common absolutes. Due to the small amount of synthetic residues that remain in the end product, absolutes are not considered of therapeutic grade, and they are recommended for perfumery and fragrance use only and not for skin and body care products.

Despite its name, an essential oil is not actually an *oil* because it does not contain fatty acids. It is not prone to rancidity, and its minute molecular makeup means that it is volatile — its constituents evaporate easily. An essential oil reacts with water much as fatty oils do, by floating to the surface, though there are a few exceptions that are denser than water and sink, such as vetiver, wintergreen, sandalwood, and patchouli. Essential oils do not dissolve in water or watery solutions (such as aloe vera juice, vinegar, or hydrosols), but they do slightly lend their scent to these liquids. They mix very well in base oils and other fatty substances, such as melted shea butter or cocoa butter, and break down moderately well in rubbing alcohol or common "drinkable" alcohols such as vodka, brandy, gin, rum, and whiskey.

Essential oils give plants their unique scents and chemical makeup, and these precious, aromatic compounds can aid in the regeneration, oxygenation, and healing of the skin. They are valuable components of therapeutic personal care formulations because, due to their minute molecular size, they easily penetrate the dermis to nourish, rejuvenate, and revitalize skin cells. In contrast, many of the heavier ingredients in face and body care products, such as base oils, waxes, and thickeners, primarily remain on the skin's surface, or perhaps penetrate it just slightly. Essential oils carry their amazing remedial properties right through the surface of the skin down to its deepest layers and into the bloodstream.

ESSENTIAL (OILS) PLANT PARTS

The following are a few examples of the plant parts from which particular oils are derived.

OIL	PLANT PART
anise and fennel	seeds
cedarwood and sandalwood	wood
chamomile, lavender, neroli, and rose	flowers
cinnamon	bark or leaves
fir, pine, and spruce	needles
frankincense and myrrh	resins
gingerroot and vetiver	roots
juniper	berries
lemon, lime, and orange	rind
lemongrass and palmarosa	grass
peppermint and spearmint	leaves

Good to Know
SMALL, BUT MIGHTY

The molecular structure of a pure plant essential oil is so compact that within minutes after inhalation and a bit longer following topical application (depending on the carrier used), the oil can be detected in your breath and in your bloodstream. Just imagine what benefits your skin will receive from the rapid absorption of these regenerative and beautifying wonders of nature!

BUYING, USING, AND STORING ESSENTIAL OILS *Tips*

Essential oils are highly concentrated forms of herbal chemical energy. Producing them is labor intensive and expensive, and they should be used with respect and caution.

BUYING

It takes approximately 250 pounds of rosemary leaves, 150 pounds of lavender buds, or 50 pounds of eucalyptus leaves to produce 1 pound of essential oil. And jasmine absolute, which retails for $600 to $800 per ounce (ouch!), requires approximately 8 million handpicked blossoms, harvested before sunrise, to produce just over 2 pounds of oil. Most essential oils, however, are not nearly as pricey! Unfortunately, some oils are poor quality, so be aware of the features of a quality product.

- **The label on an essential oil bottle should list** the common name of the plant (e.g., rosemary), its botanical name (*Rosmarinus officinalis*), and, if applicable, the variety or chemotype, denoted as "ct." (*Rosmarinus officinalis* ct. verbenon).

- **Avoid buying oil marked *perfume oil**, *fragrance oil*, *scented oil*, or *essence of*, as these indicate the contents are synthetic or a synthetic blend and are of no value therapeutically.

- **Look for descriptors such as *ethically wildcrafted**, *sustainably grown*, or *certified organic*, but keep in mind that only *certified organic* has a legal definition. Many essential oils are derived from plants that were not cultivated but responsibly wild-harvested, and for them organic certification is not possible. In other cases, the plants may have been grown under rigorous sustainability standards but were not certified organic, since organic certification is often an expensive and time-consuming process, and many smaller growers just can't afford it.

- **The descriptors *therapeutic grade**, *pharmaceutical grade*, or *aromatherapeutic grade* currently have no legal standing, but a company may use them on a product label to indicate that its essential oil is of superior quality and appropriate for therapeutic use.

- **Essential oils are highly volatile and evaporate quickly.** Place a drop on a sheet of plain paper, spread it around, and then leave it for 5 to 10 hours. A real essential oil will evaporate and leave either no stain or a very small one. A vegetable oil will leave a greasy stain.

- **Vegetable oils have a greasy feel; essential oils do not.** Rub a little vegetable oil between your fingers and notice how slippery it is. An essential oil may initially feel a bit greasy, but it's absorbed quickly or feels more like water. If the essential oil feels like vegetable oil, it has probably been diluted, and if that is the case, the label should indicate this.

USING

Essential oils are so highly concentrated that few may be used neat (undiluted) on the skin, and even then, they should only be used sparingly and as directed. Lavender, tea tree, German and Roman chamomile, rose, sandalwood, helichrysum, cardamom, frankincense, and geranium (rose geranium) are some examples that may be used neat upon the skin. Always dilute an essential oil in a base oil unless you know it's safe to use neat. Educate yourself about the properties and contraindications surrounding each essential oil before you use it.

STORING

Essential oils retain their remedial properties for several years if properly stored in a dark, dry, cool place. The exception to this is citrus, pine, and fir oils: they will remain potent for only 6 to 12 months unless refrigerated, and if refrigerated, they may keep for up to 2 years or so if not frequently opened. The longest-lasting oils, which actually improve with age, are resinous oils, such as frankincense and myrrh, and thicker oils, such as patchouli and sandalwood.

Because they can be harmful if ingested, it is advisable to store essential oils out of reach of children and pets.

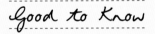

Good to Know

ESSENTIAL SAFETY

To determine potential allergic reactivity to a specific oil, combine 1 or 2 drops of the essential oil with 1 teaspoon of base oil in a small bowl. Apply a dab on the underside of your wrist, inside your upper arm, behind your ear, or behind your knee and wait 12 to 24 hours. If no irritation develops, the oil is generally safe to use.

If, while working with an essential oil, you get the oil into your eyes or nose, immediately flush the affected area with an unscented, bland fatty oil such as almond, olive, sunflower, or vegetable oil. Whole milk makes a substitute for the fatty oil in an emergency. Using plain water does not help; essential oils are attracted to fats alone. Should the pain continue or a severe headache or respiratory irritation develop, seek prompt medical attention, and take the essential oil bottle with you so the attending medical staff knows what they are dealing with.

Herbs

All civilizations, past to present, have collected herbs, prizing them for their medicinal, nutritional, flavorful, fragrant, cleansing, and skin-pampering properties and revering them for use in magical, ritual, and spiritual ceremonies.

As you try your hand at some of the recipes here, if you come across an herb that really intrigues you, my advice is to further educate yourself. Look up the plant in two or three herb books; study all its possible uses, both current and historical; learn its charms, growth habits, harvesting and storage requirements, any contraindications, and the various uses that current herbalists recommend. This additional information will augment your direct experience.

All the herbs, from flowers and leaves to seeds and roots, called for in the recipes in this book are relatively common and easy to find. If you have access to freshly grown herbs, then you may want to dry the herbs yourself. Freshly dried herbs have a wonderful just-picked aroma and vital nutrients that are at their peak — they'll simply make your products all the more delightful.

Tips
MAKING AN HERBAL INFUSION

To make a cup of herbal infusion, or herbal tea, pour 1 cup of boiling water over 1 heaping teaspoon of dried herb or 2 heaping teaspoons of fresh herb. Cover, let steep for 5 to 10 minutes (or overnight if you want a strong brew), and strain. Cool and use as directed.

Tips
HARVESTING AND DRYING HERBS

You may be surprised by how easy it is to dry many of the herbs from your garden. It's best to dry them as soon as they're picked to preserve their beneficial properties. Here are other key points to keep in mind:

- Always use a sharp knife when harvesting. Gather herbs in early to midmorning, just after any dew has dried but before the sun becomes too hot.

- Harvest flowers, such as roses, calendula, or chamomile, as soon as the bud is well formed or the flower has just opened. Lavender should always be harvested while still in bud stage.

- Harvest herbs that are free of insects and disease and have not been treated with pesticides. Herbs for harvesting should be relatively dirt-free, but if they're dusty, you can quickly rinse them in cool water and immediately pat them dry with a paper towel. To remove all dirt from harvested roots, gently scrub and then vigorously rinse them.

- Herbs can take anywhere from 4 days to 3 weeks or more to dry completely, depending upon humidity levels and the thickness of the particular botanical. When dried herbs are ready for storage, leaves will be brittle but not so dry as to shatter easily; flower petals and buds will feel dry and semicrisp or powdery; roots will be hard or ever-so-slightly pliable; and berries, bark, and seeds will be very hard and dry. Avoid overdrying herbs; it can diminish their valuable properties.

- Store dried herbs in a dark, cool, moisture-free place. Glass jars, plastic tubs, and metal tins make great storage containers. Ziplock plastic bags should only be used for temporary storage.

To dry your herbs by hanging, gather together a bundle of 5 to 10 stems (or more if the stems are ultra-slender, such as with lavender or chamomile) of a single herb and secure them together with string or rubber band around them. Hang the bundles upside down in a well-ventilated, dimly lit area where the humidity is low. Leave plenty of room between the bundles to ensure good air circulation and to keep scents from mingling.

To screen-dry your herbs, use metal or nonmetal screens or tightly stretched netting. Prepare herbs for screen drying by separating the leaves, flowers, buds, roots, berries, barks, and seed heads from the stems. Spread them in a single layer over the screen, leaving enough space between all plant parts to allow for good air circulation. If you're setting up screens outside, they should be in a partly shaded area. Cover the plant material with a single layer of cheesecloth or another screen to keep out airborne debris, feathers, pet dander, and other dirt and dust. Keep an eye on the weather, too — you don't want rain, drizzle, or fog to ruin your harvest. Soggy, moldy herbs are fodder for the compost heap.

Nut, Seed, and Grain Meal Blends

I always have a fresh supply of three "skin food" staples in my freezer: almonds, sunflower seeds, and old-fashioned rolled oats. No crafter of handmade personal care products should be without these body beautifiers. All three should be organically grown, if possible, and used in their raw form — never toasted, roasted, or salted. When a recipe calls for a particular meal, simply follow the instructions below and add the appropriate quantity to the formula you are making.

Note: Measurements are approximate due to size variations of the ingredients.

Almond meal. To make $1/2$ cup of almond meal, grind approximately 50 to 75 medium to large raw almonds (that's a heaping $1/2$ cup of whole almonds) in a blender, small food processor, or coffee grinder, using 5- to 10-second pulses, until the consistency is that of finely grated Parmesan cheese. Be careful not to overblend. Due to the high fat content of almonds, it's very easy to unintentionally end up with almond butter, especially if you're using a small grinder that generates lots of heat.

Sunflower seed meal. To make $1/2$ cup of sunflower seed meal, grind $2/3$ to $3/4$ cup of large, hulled seeds in a blender, small food processor, or coffee grinder until the consistency is that of finely grated Parmesan cheese.

Ground oatmeal. To make $1/2$ cup of ground oatmeal, grind $3/4$ to 1 cup of instant or old-fashioned rolled oats in a blender, small food processor, or coffee grinder until the consistency is somewhere between that of fine and coarse flour.

Tips
ETHICAL WILD-HARVESTING

None of the herbs listed in this book are on the endangered list, but nonetheless, when harvesting herbs in the wild (after first asking the landowner for his or her permission), never overharvest an area. Pick only what you will use immediately, leaving plenty of rootstock in the ground and fully mature, adult plants so that a new generation of seedlings will emerge during the next growing season. With the resurgence in the popularity of herbs, overharvesting of wild plants is becoming a global problem leading to the scarcity of formerly common plants. Don't contribute to this loss!

THE INGREDIENT DICTIONARY

Here is a comprehensive listing of ingredients called for in the recipes in part two. I have included information about what each ingredient can do to beautify and pamper your skin. Get to know these ingredients; they are your tools for renewed radiance, vibrance, and well-being.

ALMOND MEAL
Prunus dulcis

Cosmetic properties and uses: High in skin-pampering emollients (softening fats), the ground meal from raw almonds can be used as the base for scrubs and masks to gently exfoliate dead skin-cell buildup. Good for all skin types. With regular use, it acts as a gentle lightening agent to help even skin tone.

Possible substitute: Ground sunflower seed meal

Contraindications: To avoid further skin irritation, do not use as a scrub if skin is acneic, sensitive, sunburned, or windburned.

ALMOND MILK
Prunus dulcis

Cosmetic properties and uses: Cooling and calming to the skin. Adds a hint of creaminess to mask and scrub blends when used in lieu of water. May be used by all skin types.

ALMOND OIL, SWEET
Prunus dulcis

Cosmetic properties and uses: Pressed from the ripe kernel, this is an all-purpose, pale golden, nutritious, lightweight to medium-weight base oil, with a neutral to slightly warming energy, that can be used in a wide range of products from lotions and massage oils to body butters and balms. It

has a high fatty acid content, beneficial vitamin E, and penetrates well. Recommended for all skin types, especially dry, inflamed, or itchy skin.

Possible substitutes: Apricot or sunflower oil

ALOE
Aloe vera

Parts used: Fresh gel from the leaves or the fresh bottled juice; commercially prepared juice should be at least 99 percent pure, with less than 1 percent added oxidation and mold inhibitors.

Cosmetic properties and uses: With its cold energy and mildly astringent, anti-inflammatory, and tissue-rejuvenating properties, aloe soothes "hot" ailments such as rashes, insect bites and stings, all manner of skin burns, eczema, psoriasis, dermatitis, and blemishes. It helps restore the skin's natural pH and makes a great liquid mixing agent for mask and scrub blends. Comforting and hydrating, aloe may be used by all skin types.

APPLE
Malus domestica

Parts used: Flesh, as raw fruit purée or applesauce

Cosmetic properties and uses: The juice of the apple contains malic acid and acts as a mild astringent and gentle, nonabrasive exfoliant. Apple purée or applesauce is soothing and nourishing for acneic and sensitive skin.

APPLE CIDER VINEGAR, RAW

Cosmetic properties and uses: Contains malic acid. It can be used as a gentle, non-abrasive, exfoliating astringent (always diluted with water) for most skin types. It soothes and relieves itchy, scaly skin and restores the skin's natural pH.

Contraindications: Avoid use on very dry, sensitive, sunburned, or windburned skin.

APRICOT KERNEL OIL

Prunus armeniaca

Cosmetic properties and uses: A base oil derived from the kernel of the apricot, it has properties similar to those of almond oil, though it's a bit lighter in weight and texture. A balancing oil that penetrates readily, apricot kernel oil — particularly unrefined, organic versions — has an exquisite fruity aroma that is not to be missed. This oil is excellent for softening the delicate skin around the eyes and on the throat. It's recommended for use in eye creams and facial elixirs for oily to normal and mature skin due to its skin-tightening ability and slight astringent quality.

Possible substitutes: Almond or hazelnut oil

AVOCADO

Persea americana

Parts used: Flesh

Cosmetic properties and uses: Avocado is rich in nutritive and conditioning components such as vitamins A, B_1, B_2, and E, amino acids, lecithin, hydrating moisture, and essential fatty acids that are especially helpful to dry, chapped, irritated, and dull skin. When applied as a mask, the mashed pulp quenches the skin's thirst for both oil and water, leaving behind a soft, velvety complexion.

AVOCADO OIL

Persea americana

Cosmetic properties and uses: This full-bodied light-green base oil with a gently warming energy is derived from the fatty pulp of the fruit. Like avocado flesh, the oil is rich in nutritive and conditioning components and is beneficial to the same skin types. Due to its heavy, emollient texture, the oil takes a bit longer than other base oils to penetrate the top layer of skin. It's especially good to use in outdoor sport creams, lotions, and balms and in after-bath massage oils. Avocado oil leaves a protective barrier on the skin to help prevent moisture evaporation.

Possible substitute: Olive oil

BAKING SODA

Sodium bicarbonate

Cosmetic properties and uses: This odorless, salty-tasting white alkaline powder has skin-soothing and softening properties. It relieves the pain and itch of bee stings and rashes, deodorizes feet and underarms, and softens bathwater.

BANANA

Musa × paradisiaca

Parts used: Flesh

Cosmetic properties and uses: This nourishing fruit is used for its gentle, nonabrasive exfoliating and hydrating action in face and hand masks. It's good for all skin types, especially normal and dry.

BEESWAX

Cosmetic properties and uses: Secreted by worker honeybees, pure, unrefined, unbleached beeswax adds a sweet, honey-like fragrance and golden color to products. It is used as a thickener in creams, lotions, salves, butters, and balms. Beeswax is available in many forms: honeycomb sheets that can be broken or cut; pastilles or pellets that can be measured and melted with ease; and solid blocks and small chunks that can be placed in a ziplock freezer bag and whacked with a hammer to break up into small, measurable pieces. When melted, beeswax hardens quickly as it cools.

Possible substitutes: Refined vegetable emulsifying wax (it does not have the same aromatically alluring qualities as beeswax but is a good vegan substitute)

BLACKBERRY

Rubus villosus

Parts used: Leaves

Cosmetic properties and uses: Use as a gentle astringent ingredient for oily and normal skin.

Possible substitutes: Strawberry, sage, or raspberry leaves

BUTTERMILK

Cosmetic properties and uses: A mild, nonabrasive, bleaching exfoliant, buttermilk contains natural lactic acid, which helps dissolve the glue that binds surface dead-skin cells together, allowing them to slough off easily, leaving behind soft, evenly toned skin. I use it primarily in masks as a mixing agent. Please purchase it in organic form when available. Either whole or low-fat versions can be used.

Possible substitute: Plain organic yogurt

Contraindications: Some people with extremely irritated, hypersensitive, sunburned, or windburned skin may experience discomfort and a stinging sensation from buttermilk, but this is rare in my experience.

CALENDULA

Calendula officinalis

Parts used: Flower petals, essential oil (CO_2)

Cosmetic properties and uses: Orange calendula flowers are known for their calming, anti-inflammatory, and skin-rejuvenating properties. Both the flowers and the essential oil are slightly astringent and antiseptic, and they can be used in lotions, creams, elixirs, and balms for all skin types — especially for skin that is sensitive, environmentally damaged, acneic, irritated, or chapped. Calendula is excellent in children's formulas.

Possible flower substitute: German chamomile

CARDAMOM

Elettaria cardamomum

Parts used: Essential oil

Cosmetic properties and uses: Derived from the cardamom pod, this warming, gently stimulating oil has a soft, sweet, spicy scent with woody-citrus undertones. It blends well with other essential oils such as neroli, orange, cinnamon bark, ginger, cedarwood, and ylang ylang. For an intoxicating romantic combination, mix it with rose and vanilla essential oils.

CARROT SEED
Daucus carota
Parts used: Essential oil
Cosmetic properties and uses: This clear, rich, golden-orange essential oil has a warm, dry, woody, earthy aroma. It aids in restoring elasticity to sagging, wrinkled, or sun-damaged skin but is excellent for all skin types. Combine it with rose hip seed oil when making facial elixirs and under-eye conditioning treatments.
Contraindications: Avoid use if pregnant or breastfeeding.

CASTILE SOAP, LIQUID
Cosmetic properties and uses: This gentle soap, typically formulated with a blend of oils such as hemp, coconut, olive, castor, palm kernel, jojoba, and sunflower, can be used to bathe your entire body or as a base for herbal shampoos. If you have oily skin and prefer to use soap as your primary cleanser, this is the soap to choose. As a general rule, always dilute it by 50 percent with distilled or purified water, as castile soap is a concentrated product. I use it primarily when making herbal body wash formulations.
Contraindications: Avoid use on dry skin, scalp, and hair.

CASTOR OIL
Ricinus communis
Cosmetic properties and uses: This clear to slightly yellow, shiny, viscous base oil is processed from the seeds of an annual shrub.

It's highly emollient and particularly good for softening rough, dry heels, knees, and elbows and patches of eczema and psoriasis. When applied to nails, it imparts a protective shield against exposure to drying detergents, hot water, and winter air.

CHAMOMILE, GERMAN
Matricaria recutita
Parts used: Flowers, essential oil
Cosmetic properties and uses: This essential oil is slightly viscous and a surprisingly deep, velvety blue color with an intense, pungent, herbaceous-floral aroma. It has high levels of chamazulene and alpha-bisabolol (chemical components known for calming inflammation and soothing skin irritations), and it has a cooling energy with gentle astringency and effective antibacterial, antifungal, and antihistamine properties. Use it for treating sensitive or inflamed skin; dermatitis, eczema, psoriasis, and active acne respond well to this remedial oil. Use the pretty yellow flowers in teas, toners, lotions, and creams for all skin types.
Possible flower substitute: Calendula
Contraindications: Generally nonirritating, but may cause dermatitis in some sensitive individuals.

CHAMOMILE, ROMAN
Chamaemelum nobile, syn. *Anthemis nobilis*
Parts used: Essential oil
Cosmetic properties and uses: This oh-so-gentle golden oil, with its mild antispasmodic, relaxing, and tissue-mending properties, has an intensely sweet

fruity-floral, warm, apple-like herbaceous scent, and it is used in body balm and butter formulations to both soothe the mind and comfort irritated skin. It is gentle enough to use with very young children and blends well with other floral essential oils such as rose, lavender, ylang ylang, German chamomile, geranium, and neroli, as well as most citruses. **Contraindications:** Generally nonirritating, but may cause dermatitis in some sensitive individuals.

CINNAMON

Cinnamomum zeylanicum, C. verum
Parts used: Bark, in powdered and stick form
Cosmetic properties and uses: Use sharp, spicy, warming cinnamon powder (my favorite is Vietnamese) primarily to add fragrance to masks and scrubs. It has antiseptic properties, but only when used in amounts so great that they'd be irritating to the skin and nasal passages. Cinnamon sticks add aromatic interest to my Spicy Aftershave Tonic (page 92).
Contraindications: Avoid getting cinnamon powder into your eyes and mucous membranes — it may cause tearing, stinging, or sneezing.

CLAY, POWDERED: WHITE, GREEN, AND RED

Cosmetic properties and uses: Clay is the result of hundreds, if not thousands, of years of decay, pulverization, and compression of minerals, flora, and fauna. It's extremely mineral-rich, which is why it's so good for the skin. Various types can be used in creating masks, cleansers, and powders. Masks take advantage of clay's remarkable absorbent powers. As it dries, it actually raises the temperature of the skin, boosting circulation and encouraging the removal of toxins and excess sebum. In face or body cleansers, clay acts as a gentle exfoliant, leaving skin velvety smooth. In powders, it helps keep the skin deodorized and moisture-free.
Contraindications: Clay-based masks draw oil and moisture from the skin; avoid them if you have dry skin unless they are blended with an emollient liquid such as cream, half-and-half, coconut milk, almond milk, or full-fat yogurt. A clay-based cleanser is fine for use on dry skin, though, because it's immediately rinsed off instead of remaining on the skin to harden like a mask.

White Clay

Also referred to as *white cosmetic clay* or *white kaolin clay,* this is a very mild, fine clay that's practically pure aluminum silicate with traces of other minerals such as zinc and magnesium. It's best suited for environmentally damaged, sensitive, mature, or delicate skin, unless the skin is very dry, in which case you should blend the clay with an emollient liquid to ameliorate its drying nature (see those mentioned immediately above). White clay is so gentle that nearly anyone can use it.

Green Clay

This pale green clay, sometimes called *French green clay,* has a high concentration of chromium, nickel, and copper. It's best suited for oily and combination skin because of its strong absorptive qualities. It also works well on acneic skin, which often can't tolerate irritating chemical peels and harsh, granular exfoliants.

Red Clay

With a rusty, medium-red color, this clay has a high iron, silica, magnesium, calcium, and potassium content and is best suited for cleansing and toning normal skin.

CLOVE BUD

Eugenia caryophyllata

Parts used: Essential oil, whole cloves

Cosmetic properties and uses: Clove is spicy, warming, stimulating, and broadly antiseptic, and it is useful in skin care formulas for its fragrance and ability to fight potential infection. I use it in my recipes for aftershave, acne care, and hand and nail oils.

Contraindications: Avoid using clove essential oil if you are pregnant or breastfeeding. Always use the essential oil highly diluted, as it can be extremely irritating to the skin.

COCOA BUTTER

Theobroma cacao

Cosmetic properties and uses: Derived from the cocoa bean, this sweet, chocolate-fragranced, emollient, skin-conditioning butter is hard at room temperature but melts when applied to the skin. It lends a thick, creamy consistency to lotions, creams, body butters, balms, and some body oils, and it is a wonderful addition to recipes for after-sun care. It's completely edible and tastes like a combination of vanilla beans and chocolate.

COCONUT MILK

Cosmetic properties and uses: Aromatic milk derived from the meat of the coconut fruit is high in emollient, skin-conditioning fats. It can be used as a blending liquid, in lieu of water, when making masks for normal and dry skins. You can buy it in canned form in low-fat or full-fat versions.

COCONUT OIL

Cocos nucifera

Cosmetic properties and uses: Use only organically grown, unrefined coconut oil, sometimes called virgin coconut oil. Its sweet, exotic fragrance and smooth flavor are reminiscent of a tropical paradise. Refined coconut oil is void of both fragrance and flavor. Coconut oil is a highly emollient base oil derived from the fruit of the coconut palm and is solid at temperatures below 76°F (24°C). It's an excellent oil for all-over use, and some people swear by it as the ultimate skin softener and after-sun treatment. Use this tasty, beneficial oil in body balms, butters, and creams; cleansing creams and lotions; or any oil-based skin product from which you desire a penetrating, softening effect.

COCONUT WATER

Cosmetic properties and uses: This tasty, thirst-quenching clear liquid is found in the center of the coconut. Incredibly hydrating and lower in fat content than coconut milk, it can be used as a blending liquid, in lieu of water, when making masks for all skin types.

COMFREY

Symphytum officinale

Parts used: Root, leaves

Cosmetic properties and uses: Comfrey root, prepared as a tea, is soothing, mildly astringent, slightly mucilaginous, and emollient. To make the tea, prepare the root as a decoction: that is, simmer it for 20 minutes, then strain. Dip your fingers into the tea and notice how slippery and smooth it feels. Use it as a gentle, hydrating toner for inflamed, sensitive, environmentally damaged, or dry skin. Your skin will find this herb very comforting. I use comfrey leaves in facial steam recipes to pamper and soothe dry, irritated skin.

Possible substitute: Marshmallow root for comfrey root

CORNMEAL

Zea mays

Cosmetic properties and uses: Cornmeal is a naturally abrasive exfoliant used in body and facial scrub recipes. Purchase it in organic form when available, as most non-organic corn is genetically modified.

Contraindications: Avoid use on acneic, inflamed, sensitive, sunburned, or wind-burned skin.

CORNSTARCH

Zea mays

Cosmetic properties and uses: Common culinary cornstarch is a silky-textured, starchy flour made from corn that I use as part of the moisture-absorbent base blend for deodorant foot powders. If possible, purchase organic, as most nonorganic cornstarch is made from genetically modified corn.

CREAM, DAIRY

Cosmetic properties and uses: This fatty emollient can be used in lieu of water to mix with powdered face and body cleansers and scrub blends. It's superb for softening normal and dry skin, and it's also very soothing. You can use either light or heavy cream. Purchase it in organic form when available.

CUCUMBER

Cucumis sativus

Parts used: Fresh, peeled slices

Cosmetic properties and uses: Cucumber is incredibly hydrating for all skin types and has an amazing toning and tightening effect, perfect for soothing and reviving tired, parched skin tissue around the delicate eye area.

ELDER FLOWER

Sambucus canadensis

Parts used: Flowers

Cosmetic properties and uses: The fragrant flowers make a soothing wash for both eye and skin irritations. Good for all skin types.

Possible substitutes: Comfrey root or marshmallow root

EPSOM SALT

Magnesium sulfate

Cosmetic properties and uses: An excellent source of the muscle-relaxing mineral magnesium, this salt relieves aches and pains and helps release lactic acid buildup in overused muscles and is good for use in soaks and bath salt blends to ease sore muscles.

It's especially good for reviving dog-tired, swollen, achy feet or achy hands in foot and hand baths.

Contraindications: Consult a health professional before use if you are pregnant or breastfeeding. Avoid use on irritated, sensitive, abraded, sunburned, or windburned skin. May sting and further dehydrate already dry skin.

EUCALYPTUS
Eucalyptus radiata
Parts used: Essential oil
Cosmetic properties and uses: This essential oil, with its uplifting, slightly spicy and medicinal aroma, has powerful antiseptic capacities and can decongest and open sinuses. Eucalyptus has a warming energy, even though inhalation yields a cooling sensation. It also helps relieve sore muscles and feet. Multiple varieties of eucalyptus are available; *E. globulus* is more common, but *E. radiata* is gentler on the skin.

Contraindications: Use caution if you suffer from asthma, and do not use during an asthma attack. Do not use on or near the face of children under the age of 10, as it may be too stimulating to the central nervous system. Do not use in conjunction with homeopathic remedies.

FENNEL, SWEET
Foeniculum vulgare
Parts used: Seeds
Cosmetic properties and uses: Add sweetly fragrant, licorice-like fennel seed to facial steam blends for its gentle, cleansing, soothing, and hydrating benefit to all skin types.

A fennel-seed infusion makes an all-purpose toner or splash for everyone's skin. The seeds themselves can be chewed to freshen breath or added to aftershave blends for their slightly spicy, sweet aroma.

FRANKINCENSE
Boswellia carterii
Parts used: Essential oil (CO_2)
Cosmetic properties and uses: This oil, derived from the dried plant resin, has a heavy, complex, balsamic-woody fragrance that combines slightly sweet and warm, pungent notes and is traditionally used for perfumery and in incense blends. It is reported to reduce anxiety and tension by slowing and deepening the breath. You can also use it to rejuvenate tired, sagging skin and accelerate the healing of skin blemishes and small wounds. Frankincense is a wonderful ingredient in facial elixirs or oil blends for acneic, environmentally damaged, or mature skin.

Possible substitute: If the CO_2 extract is unavailable, the steam-distilled version is fine to use.

GERANIUM, ROSE
Pelargonium graveolens,
P. x asperum
Parts used: Essential oil
Cosmetic properties and uses: Most often you'll find this essential oil listed as simply *geranium*. Either botanical Latin name is accurate. The oil, derived from the plant's leaves, stalks, and flowers, has a muted yet tenacious, roselike, earthy-green scent and uplifting, centering, and balancing qualities, with a cooling energy. When inhaled, it helps relieve stress,

fatigue, and anxiety. It makes a good addition to facial elixirs formulated for mature, combination, or environmentally damaged skin, but because it helps balance sebum production, it can be used for all skin types.

GINGER
Zingiber officinalis

Parts used: Powdered root, essential oil
Cosmetic properties and uses: The sweet, woody-spicy, warming, softly fresh aroma of this herb is familiar, grounding, and comforting. I use the powdered root in body scrub recipes and the essential oil in body oil formulations for the fragrance and circulatory-stimulating properties it lends.

GLYCERIN, VEGETABLE

Cosmetic properties and uses: Derived from vegetable fats, this is clear, slippery, moisturizing, water-soluble, viscous, and sweet-tasting and acts as a humectant. It's a good addition to lotions and creams specifically formulated to rehydrate skin.

GRAPEFRUIT
Citrus paradisi

Parts used: Essential oil
Cosmetic properties and uses: Cold-pressed from the fruit's peel, this light, sweet-tart, refreshing essential oil with a stimulating aroma helps balance moods, lift spirits, and boost self-esteem. It has a slightly warming energy, with antibacterial, detoxifying, and astringent properties, among others. In facial elixirs it helps to relieve congested, acneic, and combination skin, improving lymph flow and remedying blemishes. I also add it to hand and nail butter formulations for the delightful fragrance — it's one of my favorites!

Contraindications: Presents a low risk of phototoxicity but is considered generally nonirritating.

HAZELNUT OIL
Corylus avellana

Cosmetic properties and uses: This is a delicate, highly penetrative base oil derived from the hazelnut that smells lovely but is not overwhelming. The cold-pressed, unrefined version has a fatty, nutty aroma and darker color than the refined oils on the market. It is gently warming and nourishing, with an astringent property that is particularly recommended for oily and combination skins.
Possible substitute: Apricot kernel oil

HELICHRYSUM
Helichrysum italicum; H. angustifolium

Parts used: Essential oil
Cosmetic properties and uses: *Helichrysum* is also known as e*verlasting* or *immortelle*. This yellow to slightly amber essential oil is steam-distilled from the plant's flowers. Highly aromatic, with warm, earthy, herbal, curry-like undertones, it has very potent anti-inflammatory, skin cell–regenerating, and antifungal properties. It's indicated as an aid in healing bruises, sprains, open wounds and cuts, acne, eczema, and psoriasis, and it is wonderful for use with environmentally damaged and mature skin. When blended with rose hip seed oil and consistently applied over time, it helps reduce the appearance of scar tissue and stretch marks.

HONEY

Cosmetic properties and uses: Sweet, sticky honey acts as a humectant. Use it in hydrating, soothing masks for all skin types. Use only raw honey; heated honey does not have the same powerful enzymatic and nutritional properties.

HYDROSOLS

Cosmetic properties and uses: Aromatic hydrosols, also known as *floral waters*, *flower waters*, *hydrolats*, *hydroflorates*, or *distillates*, have similar properties to essential oils but are far less concentrated, containing the water-soluble molecules of the essential oil in trace amounts as well as other water-soluble components of the plant. They are typically the by-product of essential oil manufacturing, but superior quality hydrosols are produced by devoted manufacturers who steam-distill small batches of fresh floral and plant material strictly to produce hydrosols. Hydrosols are especially recommended for people with ultra-sensitive, tender, or delicate skin, including the elderly and very young children, for whom even a tiny diluted amount of essential oil would be too irritating. Hydrosols can be used as facial spritzers or toners to rehydrate and freshen the skin or to cool a hot flash. They are wonderful in lotion and cream recipes and as the liquid mixing agent for clay masks. And as a bonus, you can spray them in your surroundings to energize or relax your mind.

Chamomile (*Chamaemelum nobile or Matricaria recutita*)

This soothing and balancing hydrosol is good for all skin types, especially sensitive, irritated, environmentally damaged, or mature skin. It has a floral, applelike, relaxing fragrance and acts as a gentle, calming agent for both the skin and the psyche.

Geranium, rose (*Pelargonium graveolens*)

The clean, roselike aroma of this hydrosol lifts the spirits. Slightly astringent, it balances all skin types, especially mature, combination, and environmentally damaged skin. Used as a facial spritzer, it is cooling for hot flashes. It also eliminates stale odors.

Lavender (*Lavandula angustifolia*)

This classic hydrosol has a clean, fresh fragrance that surprisingly differs from the typical sweet, soft, floral fragrance of lavender essential oil; instead it's subtle and grassy with floral undertones. Gently astringent, antiseptic, and calming, this hydrosol delivers relief to skin irritations and sunburn, but it's good for all skin types.

Possible substitute: Lavandin (*Lavandula × intermedia*)

Lemon balm (*Melissa officinalis*)

The muted lemony aroma of this hydrosol uplifts a down mood and calms mental stress. Mildly anti-inflammatory, it's beneficial and cooling when used on cold sores, herpes outbreaks, eczema, psoriasis, general dermatitis, or "angry," red, acneic skin. It can be used on all skin types, especially those in need of soothing.

Neroli (*Citrus aurantium*)

This hydrosol's delicate fragrance is reminiscent of orange blossoms and jasmine with a hint of cool green. One of my favorites, with grounding and calming qualities, it acts as a mild skin-toning astringent and assists in sebum regulation. It's beneficial to acneic, irritated, oily, sensitive, environmentally damaged, or mature skin.

Rosemary (*Rosmarinus officinalis*)

With its refreshing, energizing, herbaceous fragrance, this hydrosol acts as a stimulating, mild astringent for oily, combination, and normal skin and improves sluggish circulation. Keep a bottle in the office for an afternoon aromatic pick-me-up. Spray the surrounding air, your hair, wrists, face, and neck — it will help lift mental fog and energize your thought processes.

JOJOBA OIL
Simmondsia chinensis

Cosmetic properties and uses: A medium-textured base oil (technically a liquid wax ester) derived from pressed plant seeds or beans and chemically similar to our own emollient, protective sebum, jojoba penetrates well, leaving no oily residue. It's one of my favorite base oils for facial elixirs because it does not turn rancid and requires no refrigeration. It's also an excellent all-purpose skin lubricant for every skin type.

JUNIPER BERRY
Juniperus communis

Parts used: Essential oil

Cosmetic properties and uses: The refreshing, pungent, woody-sweet pine-needle-like fragrance of this oil, derived from the berries of the common evergreen shrub, is uplifting and stimulating during times of stress and fatigue. It can be used in facial elixirs to cleanse and balance oily, combination, and acneic skin.

Contraindications: Avoid if pregnant or if you have a kidney disorder. May be a potential skin irritant.

LAVENDER
Lavandula angustifolia

Parts used: Flower buds, essential oil

Cosmetic properties and uses: The mature buds can be made into an infusion for use as a soothing face wash or toner for all skin types, especially irritated, sensitive, and acneic skin, and I use the dried, powdered buds in facial cleanser and mask formulations.

Lavender essential oil is one of the most universally useful essential oils. It is so gentle that it can be used undiluted on the skin if applied to small areas. It has a soft, floral, herbaceous aroma that is well known for its relaxing, calming effect on the central nervous system. Sedative, antispasmodic, and antiseptic, this essential oil is a must for all first-aid kits. It can be used to relieve sunburns, insect bites, cuts, blemishes, headaches, muscular aches, painful sinuses, colds, flu, and menstrual cramps and can induce sleep in the most chronic insomniac.

LEMON
Citrus limonum

Parts used: Juice, essential oil, rind

Cosmetic properties and uses: Cold-pressed from the rind, the essential oil has a clean, sharp, bright, refreshing, citrus aroma and uplifting, stimulating, invigorating properties, with a cooling energy. The juice, when diluted, acts as a moderate astringent and disinfectant and a mild bleaching agent, benefiting imbalanced, blotchy, oily, combination, and acneic skin and helping to restore natural skin pH. Use the dried, powdered rind in face and body scrubs and the essential oil — sparingly — in face cleansers, astringents, elixirs, foot scrubs and baths, nail conditioning oils, and body lotions.

Possible substitutes: Tangerine juice for its astringent property; dried, powdered orange rind can be substituted for lemon rind

Contraindications: Use lemon essential oil in moderation and always highly diluted, as it is a potential skin irritant. May cause photosensitivity to skin exposed to sunlight and/or tanning beds within 12 hours of use.

LEMON BALM
Melissa officinalis
Parts used: Leaves
Cosmetic properties and uses: Lemon balm, a member of the mint family, has a lovely, soft, lemony-herbaceous scent and a cooling energy. It acts as a sedative, antidepressant, nervine, mild astringent, anti-inflammatory, and antiviral. The uplifting fragrance is said to make the heart joyful. In this book, I use the leaves in mild astringents for oily, acneic, combination, and normal skin, but because it is so gentle, it can be enjoyed by all skin types.

LEMONGRASS
Cymbopogon citratus
Parts used: Leaves, essential oil

Cosmetic properties and uses: Lemongrass, with its stimulating, pungent, earthy, lemony scent, has astringent, antiviral, antifungal, antibacterial, and deodorizing properties. Both the essential oil and an infusion made from the leaves can be used in creams, lotions, and skin cleansers formulated for normal, combination, oily, and acneic skin. I also like to add lemongrass to foot powder recipes for its clean, fresh, purifying scent.

Contraindications: Avoid the essential oil if you are pregnant or taking multiple medications. May be a potential skin irritant on sensitive skin.

MACADAMIA NUT OIL
Macadamia integrifolia
Cosmetic properties and uses: This light-to medium-thick, penetrating base oil has a slightly nutty aroma — if unrefined — and high levels of monounsaturated fatty acids as well as ample vitamin E. Like jojoba oil, it has a chemical makeup that closely resembles that of sebum. Use it in facial elixirs for mature or environmentally damaged skin and skin that's irritated, sunburned, or windburned. It's often used in blends to help soften scar tissue.

MARSHMALLOW
Althaea officinalis
Parts used: Root
Cosmetic properties and uses: The Greek word *althaea* means "to heal." Marshmallow root contains a soothing mucilage that, when steeped in simmering water, produces a slippery, remedial goo that is quite beneficial for weather-beaten, chapped, or sun-damaged

skin. It's good for all skin types, but especially those needing added moisture and comfort for irritated tissues.

Possible substitute: Comfrey root

MILK

Cosmetic properties and uses: Milk contains skin-softening lipids and mildly exfoliating lactic acid. It makes a pampering liquid additive for normal, dry, and sensitive skin when used in powdered masks, facial scrubs, and body cleansers. Purchase organic milk (whole or low-fat) when available.

MYRRH

Commiphora myrrha

Parts used: Essential oil

Cosmetic properties and uses: Derived by steam-distilling the crude oleoresin that exudes from the trunk of this desert-dwelling tree native to northeast Africa and areas of Arabia adjacent to the Red Sea, myrrh essential oil is generally an amber-colored, semiviscous liquid with a warm, heavy, slightly musty, earthy balsamic aroma. Having skin-tightening, antifungal, anti-inflammatory, antibacterial, and tissue-mending properties, it is valued for use in facial creams, lotions, and elixirs for all skin types but especially environmentally damaged and mature skin. Makes a remedial addition to hand and nail butters and oils.

Contraindications: Avoid if you are pregnant or breastfeeding.

MYRTLE, GREEN

Myrtus communis

Parts used: Essential oil

Cosmetic properties and uses: Derived from myrtle's twigs, leaves, and flowers, the essential oil has a fragrance similar to that of fresh, camphorous eucalyptus, but it is softer and more delicate, with a warming energy. It's used on oily, combination, or acneic skin for its antiseptic and astringent actions. May also be used in formulations for mature skin as it contracts and tones tissue. The aroma is said to quell anger, calm emotional upset, and lift a down mood.

Contraindications: Avoid if you are pregnant or breastfeeding or if you are taking multiple medications.

NEROLI

Citrus aurantium

Parts used: Essential oil

Cosmetic properties and uses: This is one of my favorite essential oils, steam-distilled from the flowers of the Seville (bitter) orange tree. Gentle to the skin and soothing to the psyche, it has a rich, erotic, delicate, yet tenacious orange-blossom aroma and cooling energy. It can be used on all skin types but is especially beneficial to mature and environmentally damaged skin. Use it in facial elixirs to promote cell regeneration and improve elasticity. It blends well with other floral, citrus, and woody essential oils.

NUTMEG

Myristica fragrans

Parts used: Ground seed

Cosmetic properties and uses: A familiar, warm, potent, and gently stimulating spice with a rich, sweet, piney-woody aroma. I primarily use it in body polish formulas made with sugar to add a delicious, comforting fragrance.

Contraindications: Avoid if you are pregnant or breastfeeding.

OATMEAL
Avena sativa

Cosmetic properties and uses: Soothing to all types of skin irritations and sensitivities, finely ground oatmeal makes a gentle abrasive base for face and body scrubs, powdered cleansers, masks, and bath bags.

Possible substitute: Oat flour

OLIVE OIL, EXTRA-VIRGIN
Olea europaea

Cosmetic properties and uses: This rich, moderately heavy green base oil is derived from the first pressing of green or ripe olives. It has a moderately strong olive aroma, high levels of monounsaturated fats, and beneficial vitamins and minerals. If you purchase oil of superior quality, it's also packed with valuable antioxidants — a true beauty boost for your skin. Olive oil can be blended with a lighter-textured, odorless base oil in body care products, if you desire. It's wonderful as a makeup remover and skin softener, though completely masking its fragrance can be difficult if you are using lighter-scented essential oils. When color and fragrance aren't a concern, however, such as in medicinal salves, many herbalists use it exclusively. Personally, I don't mind the scent, as I know that the oil's inherent skin-conditioning properties are wonderful for the health and vitality of my dry, mature skin. Used alone, it makes an excellent conditioning oil for dry

nails and feet and patches of dry eczema and psoriasis.

Possible substitutes: Avocado or jojoba oil

ORANGE, SWEET
Citrus sinensis

Parts used: Dried rind, essential oil

Cosmetic properties and uses: The ground dried peel of this familiar fruit has a neutral to warming energy and is often used in aromatic body scrubs. The sweet, fruity essential oil, cold-pressed from the rind, is used in cleansing creams and lotions for oily, combination, and normal skin for its gentle astringent, toning action and antibacterial properties. I love to add it to body scrubs, butters, balms, deodorizing foot formulations, and products for the hands. It adds such an amazing scent! The aroma has an uplifting yet calming effect and helps relieve anxiety.

Possible substitute: Tangerine essential oil for its astringent and fragrant properties

Contraindications: Presents a low risk of phototoxicity.

PAPAYA
Carica papaya

Parts used: Fresh, raw mashed pulp or juice

Cosmetic properties and uses: Papaya contains papain, a protein-digesting enzyme that helps "eat" or break down the dead outer layer of skin, revealing the new, fresh, smooth layer underneath. Use papaya when making masks for almost any skin type, but particularly for skin that's in need of deep cleansing, brightening, and balancing of uneven coloration. It really helps rid skin of a blotchy appearance.

Contraindications: Avoid use on irritated, sensitive, sunburned, or windburned skin.

PARSLEY
Petroselinum sativum

Parts used: Leaves

Cosmetic properties and uses: A parsley infusion is gently astringent and soothing for those who suffer from weeping or active acne, eczema, psoriasis, or any irritable dermatitis.

PEACH
Prunus persica

Parts used: Fresh, raw mashed pulp or juice

Cosmetic properties and uses: Nourishing, moisturizing, and toning for all skin types, peach also has a yummy fruity fragrance. Mix the pulp or juice with heavy cream or coconut milk for a super-emollient, hydrating, dry-skin-pampering mask.

PEPPERMINT
Mentha piperita

Parts used: Leaves, essential oil

Cosmetic properties and uses: Peppermint is a true multipurpose herb. An infusion of the leaves — cooling, deodorizing, stimulating, astringent, and antiseptic — is good for oily to normal, combination, and acneic skin. The crushed dried leaves are often added to facial scrubs and steams. The essential oil is commonly used in cooling body lotions and creams, as well as in recipes for cleansing and reviving the feet. When its aroma is inhaled, it energizes and awakens the mind. It also makes a terrific room freshener.

Possible substitutes: Spearmint leaves and essential oil, though they're not as strong in fragrance or action

Contraindications: Use in moderation; may cause sensitization in some individuals due to the menthol concentration. Do not use in conjunction with homeopathic remedies. Do not use on or near the face of children under 10, as it has a low risk of irritating the mucous membranes.

PINEAPPLE
Ananas comosus

Parts used: Fresh raw juice strained from the mashed pulp

Cosmetic properties and uses: Containing bromelain, a protein-digesting enzyme, pineapple juice aids in breaking down dead surface skin cells so that they slough off easier, resulting in softer, smoother skin. It works like papaya (page 228). Use the astringent juice in facial masks for all skin types, particularly those in need of brightening, gentle bleaching, and deep cleansing.

Contraindications: Avoid use on sensitive, sunburned, windburned, or irritated skin.

POTATO, WHITE
Solanum tuberosum

Parts used: Fresh peeled slices

Cosmetic properties and uses: Thin white potato slices are cooling and hydrating for all skin types and deliver a toning and tightening effect, perfect for soothing and reviving tired, parched skin tissue around the delicate eye area.

RASPBERRY, RED
Rubus idaeus

Parts used: Leaves, freshly pressed and strained fruit juice

Cosmetic properties and uses: The leaves have similar properties as blackberry and strawberry leaves and make an infusion that is gently astringent. Good for oily, combination, acneic, and normal skin, the fresh fruit juice contains lactic acid and, when applied to the skin, both brightens skin tone and acts as a nonabrasive exfoliant, aiding the removal of dead-skin buildup.

Possible substitutes: Strawberry or blackberry leaves or fresh strawberry juice

Contraindications: Avoid use of the fresh juice if skin is sensitive, irritated, sunburned, or windburned.

ROSE OTTO
Rosa damascena

Parts used: Petals, essential oil

Cosmetic properties and uses: Rose otto — real rose essential oil — is very expensive yet exquisite, with a deep, complex, slightly spicy, warm, true rose aroma. Valued as a skin cell regenerator, gentle antiseptic, mild astringent, mood elevator, and aphrodisiac, this oil is used in formulas for all skin types, especially mature, sensitive, and environmentally damaged skin. The dried petals (*R. damascena* and also *R. gallica* and *R. centifolia* species) are generally dark pink or deep red in color; they are powdered for use in face cleanser recipes and used whole in facial steams.

ROSE HIP SEED OIL
Rosa rubiginosa

Cosmetic properties and uses: Sometimes called *rosa mosqueta* oil, this is a medium-weight, pale, orange-red base oil derived from the seeds of the Andean rose hip. When very fresh, it has a light, tart aroma. High in essential fatty acids, it's a superior facial and body care oil for mature, environmentally damaged, prematurely aged, and devitalized skin. Use this oil combined with tamanu (page 232) in facial elixirs and creams specifically to rejuvenate and soften skin damaged by scars, stretch marks, and extreme weather exposure. **Note:** This oil is fragile and requires refrigeration. It will keep for only 6 months.

Contraindications: Avoid use on oily, acneic, or combination skin; this oil may further exacerbate these conditions.

ROSEMARY
Rosmarinus officinalis

Parts used: Leaves, essential oil (ct. verbenon)

Cosmetic properties and uses: The verbenon chemotype of essential oil (as opposed to the camphor and cineol chemotypes or the commonly available non-chemotype-specific rosemary essential oil) is the preferred variety for skin care, with its crisp lemony-herbaceous aroma, less heating energy, and surprisingly sedative effects. Use it in facial elixirs for toning oily to normal and combination skin and for its cell-regenerating and antiseptic properties. It makes a good addition to hand and nail care balms and oils and deodorizing foot treatments. It also helps open clogged sinuses and mend wounds. The dried, resinous leaves are often included in facial scrubs, steams, and toners.

Contraindications: Avoid use of all varieties of rosemary essential oil if you are pregnant. Take care using any variety of rosemary essential oil on children under the age of 10, as it may be too stimulating to the respiratory system, though the verbenon chemotype is generally considered safe for children over the age of 2.

SAGE
Salvia officinalis
Parts used: Leaves
Cosmetic properties and uses: This multipurpose plant has a classic pungent, warm, herbal, spicy, "Thanksgiving" scent. The infusion is used as an astringent and antiseptic for oily, combination, acneic, and normal skin and as a disinfectant for minor cuts, abrasions, and insect bites.
Possible substitute: Strong rosemary infusion

SEA SALT
Cosmetic properties and uses: Sea salt is remedial and drying to open sores, cuts, scrapes, bug bites, dermatitis, eczema, psoriasis, and pimples. (You may have noticed how quickly blemishes or minor cuts heal after you swim in the ocean.) Use finely ground sea salt in body and foot scrub recipes as an abrasive exfoliant to slough away rough skin.
Contraindications: Do not use if your skin is dry, sensitive, or irritated in any way. Also, sea salt is much too abrasive for the face area; use only on the body, and *do not* use on skin that has been shaved within 48 hours.

SESAME OIL
Sesamum indicum
Cosmetic properties and uses: Pressed from sesame seeds, this clear, pale- to golden-yellow, antioxidant-rich base oil has a distinct aroma and small amounts of vitamins B_6 and E, plus the minerals copper, calcium, magnesium, and zinc. It's stable, with a long shelf life, though I still prefer to refrigerate it and use it within 1 year. It has a low natural SPF and thus can be used in natural sunscreen recipes. It also makes a penetrating, relaxing body and massage oil and is recommended for use on normal to dry skin. **Note:** Do not use the toasted variety of sesame oil in your skin care recipes, or else your products will manifest an "essence of stir-fry" aroma!
Possible substitutes: Sunflower seed, avocado, or olive oil

SHEA BUTTER
Butyrospermum parkii
Cosmetic properties and uses: Derived from the pressed nuts of the karite tree, in its unrefined form shea butter is a soft, cream-colored substance with a distinctive fragrance that's difficult to mask. If the scent displeases you, then purchase the white refined butter. It will be firmer but will have virtually the same properties. (I actually prefer shea butter in the refined form because I like the aromas of any added essential oils to stand out.) Shea butter is a skin-softening additive in lotions, creams, body, hand, foot balms, and after-sun products. It can even be used alone if desired.

STRAWBERRY
Fragaria vesca

Parts used: Leaves, mashed fruit pulp, juice

Cosmetic properties and uses: An infusion of strawberry leaves makes a gentle astringent or body splash for oily, combination, acneic, and normal skin. Use the fresh-pressed juice in masks for the same skin types or apply it directly onto pimples as a remedial drying aid. It contains a gentle, exfoliating acid that helps rid skin of dead-cell buildup.

Possible substitutes: Blackberry or raspberry leaves or fresh raspberry fruit

SUGAR

Cosmetic properties and uses: Sugar can be used as an abrasive exfoliant just like sea salt in body and foot scrub recipes, but because it doesn't dry or sting the skin, many people prefer it over salt. Sugar contains natural glycolic acids, meaning it also exfoliates on a chemical level, rather than by abrasion alone. Purchase organic sugar, if available. You can use white or brown sugar, in finely granulated form.

Contraindications: Avoid use on abraded, irritated, sunburned, windburned, or sensitive skin or skin that has been shaved within 48 hours. Sugar is too abrasive to be used on the face; use only on the body.

SUNFLOWER SEED MEAL
Helianthus annuus

Cosmetic properties and uses: Rich in lubricating lipids and nutrients, the ground meal of hulled raw sunflower seeds makes a gentle, emollient base for scrubs and masks for normal and dry skin. Because of its high fat content and the softness of its granules, it can be used to exfoliate even sensitive and acneic skin, but always use a gentle touch.

Possible substitute: Almond meal, if very finely ground

Contraindications: Do not use on irritated, sunburned, or windburned skin.

SUNFLOWER SEED OIL
Helianthus annuus

Cosmetic properties and uses: This light- to medium-textured, clear to pale yellow base oil is pressed from sunflower seeds and rich in essential fatty acids, lecithin, minerals, and vitamin E. Deeply nourishing and conditioning, with a cooling energy, it is good for all skin types and penetrates readily. It is an inexpensive all-purpose oil that may be used in all lotion and cream recipes. Always purchase organic when available, as nearly all of the sunflower oil commercially available is chock-full of synthetic chemical residues.

Possible substitute: Almond oil

TAMANU OIL
Calophyllum inophyllum

Cosmetic properties and uses: This rich brownish-green base oil is also known as *calophyllum* or *foraha oil*. Derived from the ripened seeds of a native Tahitian tree, it has a sweet, earthy fragrance reminiscent of buttercream frosting or Kahlúa. It's analgesic, antibacterial, and anti-inflammatory. Use it in oil blends specifically formulated to help fade scars, heal burns, and soothe chapped skin, eczema, psoriasis, and shingles. It's a perfect choice for environmentally damaged, mature, or very dry skin.

TANGERINE

Citrus reticulata

Parts used: Essential oil

Cosmetic properties and uses: Derived from the cold-pressed peel, this oil has a tart, sweet, fresh, and uplifting aroma that's calming and soothing to the psyche. It's nearly identical in therapeutic properties to sweet orange and may be used as a substitute for that oil.

Possible substitute: Sweet orange essential oil

Contraindications: Presents a low risk of phototoxicity.

TEA TREE

Melaleuca alternifolia

Parts used: Essential oil

Cosmetic properties and uses: This essential oil, derived from the leaves of the melaleuca tree, has a strong camphorous, slightly spicy, balsamic, medicinal odor. It is very safe and a potent antibacterial, antifungal, and antiviral agent. It makes an excellent addition to the home medicine chest. It helps heal acne, open wounds, cuts, infections, rashes, and dermatitis and works well in cleansers, astringents, facial elixirs, and masks for acneic and blemish-prone skin. It can be used neat as a spot treatment for pimples.

Contraindications: Potentially sensitizing in some individuals if used undiluted, but generally considered nonirritating.

THYME

Thymus vulgaris

Parts used: Essential oil (ct. linalool), leaves

Cosmetic properties and uses: Derived from thyme's leaves and flowering tops, the linalool chemotype of thyme essential oil is skin-friendly and gentle, unlike red thyme (ct. thymol) or the commonly available non-chemotype-specific thyme essential oil, both of which can be hot and irritating to the skin and mucous membranes. It has a sweet, warm, herbaceous, lightly medicinal aroma and is a wonderfully effective antibacterial, antifungal, and antiviral agent. It's quite remedial for weeping or active acne and rashes resulting from poison oak, poison ivy, and sumac or general contact dermatitis. Use it in cleansers, astringents, lotions, facial elixirs, and masks for acneic and blemish-prone skin. An infusion of thyme leaves produces an astringent liquid that can be used for an oily, combination, or normal complexion or as a cleansing wound wash.

Possible substitute: Tea tree essential oil, though it has a much more penetrating, medicinal odor

VANILLA

Vanilla planifolia

Parts used: Essential oil (CO_2 extract or absolute)

Cosmetic properties and uses: The essential oil has a familiar sweet, rich, warm, creamy fragrance and is derived from the vanilla bean. It balances mood and reduces stress, is a calming aphrodisiac, and softens all fragrance blends. Vanilla is one of my favorite scents, and I use the essential oil in body creams and butters.

VITAMIN E OIL
D-alpha-tocopherol or mixed tocopherols

Cosmetic properties and uses: This antioxidant oil acts as a preservative when added to base oils, lotions, balms, body butters, and creams by preventing rancidity of fatty ingredients. When applied topically, it aids in the prevention of scar tissue. When formulating an oil-based product, I add 1,000 IU of vitamin E oil to each cup of base oil or at least 200 IU per 1/4 cup. Always purchase organic if available, as vitamin E oil is frequently extracted from sunflower seeds and soybeans grown with synthetic chemicals. Most soybeans are also genetically modified. The most convenient form to use is liquid capsules, which are generally available in 200, 400, 600, and 1,000 IU doses (check the packaging to determine how many IUs are in each capsule). Just pierce the capsule skin and squeeze out the liquid contents.

Contraindications: Because it may irritate eyes and sensitive skin, use this viscous heavy oil on the body alone, not on the face area.

VODKA

Cosmetic properties and uses: Commonly derived from the fermentation of potatoes or grains, this fragrance-free alcohol can be used as an extractive solvent in alcohol-based herbal toners and astringents for oily, combination, acneic, and normal skin and in aftershave formulas. Always purchase vodka that's 80 or 100 proof.

Contraindications: Avoid applying to dry, irritated, sensitive, sunburned, windburned, or abraded skin.

WATER

Cosmetic properties and uses: When making personal care products that call for water, always use either distilled or purified water. Distilled water is void of bacteria and will not introduce contaminants into your products. Purified water has been put through a filter to reduce minerals such as copper, chlorine, fluoride, cadmium, mercury, zinc, and arsenic. The purifying process improves taste and diminishes the likelihood that the water will negatively react with pipes, food, and, in this case, homemade skin care products. It is not totally void of bacteria, though, but is considered cleaner than tap water, which should not be used in skin care products (unless it is the only water source available) because it often contains added chemicals like chlorine and fluoride, especially if it comes from a public water utility, and waterborne bacteria. If you must use tap water, boil it first. I generally use purified bottled water or filtered water for many recipes calling for water, such as herbal facial steams, masks, scrubs, liquid soap blends, herbal toners and astringents, but for my cleansing creams, lotions, body creams, and butters, I prefer distilled water to minimize the potential for mold formation in products that are a blend of watery ingredients and fats.

WHEAT GERM
Triticum aestivum

Cosmetic properties and uses: Wheat germ is the heart of the wheat kernel. Due to its high fat content, it becomes rancid quickly if stored at room temperature, so look for fresh, raw wheat germ. It usually can be found in the refrigerator or freezer section of your local health food store. If you don't find wheat germ in either place, leave it on the shelf! Fresh wheat germ is rich in protein, essential fatty acids, vitamins B and E, and soluble dietary fiber. Use it in nourishing, softening facial masks for normal to very dry, environmentally damaged, and mature skin. It's especially good for sensitive, irritated, sunburned, and windburned complexions. Purchase organic wheat germ when available, as wheat is often treated with pesticides and herbicides.

WITCH HAZEL
Hamamelis virginiana

Parts used: Commercially prepared liquid

Cosmetic properties and uses: You can make your own witch hazel astringent, but the commercial version is convenient and effective. It consists primarily of water with added witch hazel alcohol extract — derived from the bark of the witch hazel tree — and acts as a gentle, nearly unscented astringent for oily, combination, acneic, and normal skin.

Contraindications: Avoid use on dry, sensitive, sunburned, or windburned skin.

YARROW
Achillea millefolium

Parts used: Leaves, flowers

Cosmetic properties and uses: Yarrow has strong anti-inflammatory, antiseptic, astringent, and styptic properties. The herbal infusion has a cooling, constricting energy and makes a potent astringent for oily, acneic, combination, and normal skin. It also makes a remedial wash for all kinds of wounds and sores.

Contraindications: Avoid use on dry or dehydrated skin. Extended use may irritate sensitive skin.

YLANG YLANG
Cananga odorata

Parts used: Essential oil

Cosmetic properties and uses: Steam-distilled from the large golden-yellow flowers of the tropical cananga tree, the tenacious, intensely sweet and spicy-floral scent of this essential oil rivals rose and jasmine oils as one of the most exotic aromas on earth. The scent is deeply tranquilizing, relaxes muscles as well as the central nervous system, balances mood, calms the mind, and acts as an antidepressant. The oil also helps regulate sebum production for all skin types. Use it in body balms and butters and facial creams. It blends well with citrus, spice, floral, and cedarwood essential oils. When you're feeling anxious, inhale ylang ylang oil directly from the bottle or apply it to pulse points.

Contraindications: May irritate sensitive skin.

YOGURT, PLAIN

Cosmetic properties and uses: A mild, non-abrasive, skin-brightening exfoliant, yogurt contains natural lactic acid, which helps dissolve the glue that binds surface dead-skin cells together, allowing them to slough off easily and leaving behind soft, evenly toned skin. It can be used alone as a skin-softening mask for all skin types or as a thick mixing liquid for powdered facial masks and scrubs. Purchase organic yogurt when available. Look for products processed with only low heat, if you can, but pasteurized yogurt will work fine.

Contraindications: Some people with extremely irritated, hypersensitive, sunburned, or windburned skin may experience slight discomfort and a mild stinging sensation from the lactic acid that naturally occurs in yogurt. Most of the time, yogurt counteracts the pain induced from environmental skin damage and helps speed healing of the condition.

ZINC OXIDE

Cosmetic properties and uses: While zinc itself is a metallic element found in nature, zinc oxide is not naturally occurring but rather created when zinc is chemically heated and combined with oxygen molecules. The two elements are vaporized, condensed, and formed into a fine crystallized white powder with anti-inflammatory, antiseptic, astringent, and skin-mending properties. Zinc oxide sits on top of the skin, providing a protective layer that helps prevent inflammatory dermatitis, itching, fungal proliferation, and odor. I primarily use it in deodorizing foot powder formulations.

Contraindications: Do not use on skin that is extremely dry, cracked, or fissured.

METRIC CONVERSION CHARTS

Unless you have finely calibrated equipment, conversions between US standard measurements and metric measurements will be somewhat inexact. It's important to convert the measurements for all ingredients in a recipe to maintain the same proportions as the original.

GENERAL FORMULA FOR METRIC CONVERSION

TO CONVERT	TO	MULTIPLY
ounces	grams	ounces by 28.35
teaspoons	milliliters	teaspoons by 4.93
tablespoons	milliliters	tablespoons by 14.79
fluid ounces	milliliters	fluid ounces by 29.57
cups	milliliters	cups by 236.59
cups	liters	cups by 0.24
quarts	milliliters	quarts by 946.36
quarts	liters	quarts by 0.946
gallons	liters	gallons by 3.785

APPROXIMATE METRIC EQUIVALENTS BY VOLUME

US	Metric
1 teaspoon	5 milliliters
1 tablespoon	15 milliliters
¼ cup	60 milliliters
½ cup	120 milliliters
1 cup	240 milliliters
1¼ cups	300 milliliters
1½ cups	355 milliliters
2 cups	480 milliliters
3 cups	710 milliliters
4 cups (1 quart)	0.95 liter
4 quarts (1 gallon)	3.8 liters

RESOURCES

THE ANANDA APOTHECARY
888-758-6360
www.anandaapothecary.com
Therapeutic-grade essential oils and blends, hydrosols, aromatherapy supplies, carrier oils, bottles, essential oil diffusers, and books

AROMATHERAPEUTIX
800-308-6284
www.aromatherapeutix.com
Huge variety of essential oils and oil blends, bottles, soaps, herbal body and health care products, essential oil diffusers, and more

AROMATICS INTERNATIONAL
406-273-9833
www.aromatics.com
Organic and wildcrafted essential oils and oil blends, hydrosols, carrier oils, essential oil accessories, and packaging

AURA CACIA
FRONTIER NATURAL PRODUCTS CO-OP
844-550-7200
www.auracacia.com
Essential oils, base oils, and natural skin and body care products

EDEN BOTANICALS
707-509-0041
www.edenbotanicals.com
Wholesale essential oils, CO_2 extracts, and absolutes for aromatherapy, natural perfumery, and body and facial care; superior quality

FRONTIER NATURAL PRODUCTS CO-OP
844-550-6200
www.frontiercoop.com
Large inventory of essential oils, base oils, organic herbs, spices, cosmetic clays, beeswax, and natural body care products

HEALTHY HARVEST, LLC
www.healthyharvests.com
Best olive oil ever! Single estate/varietal, organic; exquisite aromatherapeutic facial oil blends formulated by Stephanie Tourles

JEAN'S GREENS
518-479-0471
www.jeansgreens.com
A wide range of wonderful herb products, teas, loose herbs and spices, essential oils, beeswax, butters, cosmetic clays, books, and more

MOUNTAIN ROSE HERBS
800-879-3337
www.mountainroseherbs.com
Organic bulk herbs, spices, teas, essential and base oils, packaging supplies, herbal health aids, natural personal care products, and more

NYR ORGANIC
STEPHANIE TOURLES, INDEPENDENT
CONSULTANT/LICENSED ESTHETICIAN
207-326-5009
http://us.nyrorganic.com/shop/herbs
Beautiful essential oil blends and single essential oils; exquisite organic products for skin, body, hair, and bath; herb teas; chemical-free home fragrance; organic body perfumes; essential oil diffusers; nutritional supplements; and more

ORIGINAL SWISS AROMATICS
415-479-9120
www.originalswissaromatics.com
Superior quality, authentic and genuine, organic and wildcrafted essential oils, plus facial, massage, and body care oils, hydrosols, and natural perfumes

SIMPLERS BOTANICALS
NUTRAMARKS
800-229-2512
www.simplers.com
Superior quality, therapeutic-grade, organic and wildcrafted essential oils, hydrosols, natural perfume oils, infused herbal oils, herbal extracts, and more

SKS BOTTLE & PACKAGING, INC.
518-880-6980
www.sks-bottle.com
Glass and plastic bottles, jars, and tins of all sizes

SPECIALTY BOTTLE
206-382-1100
www.specialtybottle.com
Glass and plastic bottles, jars, and tins of every size imaginable

STILLPOINT AROMATICS
928-301-8699
www.stillpointaromatics.com
Exceptional quality essential oils, aromatherapy kits, hydrosols, flower essences, carrier oils, infused oils, books, and more

RECOMMENDED READING

This list includes sources consulted for this book, as well as selections from my personal library.

Alt, Carol. *Eating in the Raw: A Beginner's Guide to Getting Slimmer, Feeling Healthier, and Looking Younger the Raw-Food Way.* Clarkson Potter, 2004.

Balch, Phyllis A. *Prescription for Nutritional Healing,* fifth edition. Revised and updated by Stacey Bell, DSC. Penguin Group, 2010.

Cousin, Pierre Jean. *Facelift at Your Fingertips: An Aromatherapy Massage Program for Healthy Skin and a Younger Face.* Storey Publishing, 2000.

Duke, James A. *The Green Pharmacy: Anti-Aging Prescriptions.* Rodale, 2001.

Fairley, Josephine, and Sarah Stacey. *Feel Fabulous Forever: The Anti-Aging Health and Beauty Bible.* Overlook Press, 1999.

Falconi, Dina. *Earthly Bodies and Heavenly Hair: Natural and Healthy Personal Care for Every Body.* Ceres Press, 1998.

Furjanic, Sheila, and Jacqueline Flynn, editors. *Milady's Art and Science of Nail Technology,* revised edition. Milady Publishing, 1992.

Gerson, Joel. *Milady's Standard Textbook for Professional Estheticians,* eighth edition. Thomson Learning, 1999.

Gladstar, Rosemary. *Herbal Healing for Women.* Simon and Schuster, 1993.

———. *Herbs for Longevity and Well-Being.* Storey Books, 1999.

———. *Rosemary Gladstar's Family Herbal: A Guide to Living Life with Energy, Health, and Vitality.* Storey Publishing, 2001.

———. *Rosemary Gladstar's Medicinal Herbs: A Beginner's Guide.* Storey Publishing, 2012.

Hampton, Aubrey, and Susan Hussey. *The Take Charge Beauty Book: The Natural Guide to Beautiful Hair and Skin.* Organica Press, 2000.

James, Kat. *The Truth about Beauty: Transform Your Looks and Your Life from the Inside Out.* Beyond Words Publishing, 2003.

Keville, Kathi, and Mindy Green. *Aromatherapy: A Complete Guide to the Healing Art,* second edition. Crossing Press, 2009.

Kloss, Jethro. *Back to Eden.* Woodbridge Press, 1939.

Lust, John B. *The Herb Book.* Bantam Books, 1974.

Maria, Donna. *Making Aromatherapy Creams and Lotions: 101 Natural Formulas to Revitalize and Nourish Your Skin.* Storey Publishing, 2000.

Ody, Penelope. *The Complete Medicinal Herbal.* Dorling Kindersley, 1993.

Phillips, Nancy, and Michael Phillips. *The Village Herbalist: Sharing Plant Medicines with Family and Community.* Chelsea Green, 2001.

Purcheron, Nerys, and Lora Cantele. *The Complete Aromatherapy and Essential Oils Handbook for Everyday Wellness.* Robert Rose, Inc., 2014.

Sachs, Melanie. *Ayurvedic Beauty Care: Ageless Techniques to Invoke Natural Beauty.* Lotus Press, 1994.

Schneider, Anny. *Wild Medicinal Plants.* Stackpole Books, 2002.

Soule, Deb. *A Woman's Book of Herbs.* Carol, 1998.

———. *How to Move Like a Gardener: Planting and Preparing Medicines from Plants.* SteinerBooks, 2013.

Tisserand, Robert, and Rodney Young. *Essential Oil Safety,* second edition. Churchill Livingstone Elsevier, 2014.

Tourles, Stephanie. *Hands-on Healing Remedies: 150 Recipes for Herbal Balms, Salves, Oils, Liniments, and Other Topical Therapies.* Storey Publishing, 2012.

———. *Making Love Potions: 64 All-Natural Recipes for Irresistible Herbal Aphrodisiacs.* Storey Publishing, 2016.

———. *Natural Foot Care: Herbal Treatments, Massage, and Exercises for Healthy Feet.* Storey Publishing, 1998.

———. *Naturally Bug-Free: 75 Nontoxic Recipes for Repelling Mosquitoes, Ticks, Fleas, Ants, Moths, and Other Pesky Insects.* Storey Publishing, 2016.

———. *Organic Body Care Recipes: 175 Homemade Herbal Formulas for Glowing Skin and a Vibrant Self.* Storey Publishing, 2007.

———. *Raw Energy: 124 Raw Food Recipes for Energy Bars, Smoothies, and Other Snacks to Supercharge Your Body.* Storey Publishing, 2009.

———. *Raw Energy in a Glass: 126 Nutrition-Packed Smoothies, Green Drinks, and Other Satisfying Raw Beverages to Boost Your Well-Being.* Storey Publishing, 2014.

Weinberg, Norma Pasekoff. *Natural Hand Care: Herbal Treatments and Simple Techniques for Healthy Hands and Nails.* Storey Publishing, 1998.

Worwood, Valerie Ann. *The Complete Book of Essential Oils and Aromatherapy,* 25th anniversary edition. New World Library, 2016.

Acknowledgments

To all the gardeners, herbalists, aromatherapists, biologists, landscapers, farmers, cosmetic chemists, elders of the past, and even the plants themselves, my lifelong teachers of the green world who have shared their wisdom with me over the years; without you, this book would have been impossible and my green soul would be unfulfilled.

I am also eternally grateful to those of you who have been my cosmetic "guinea pigs" over the years — friends, family members, and even complete strangers who allowed me to apply new personal-care concoctions to your faces, arms, legs, hands, feet, backs, and hair, and who gave me in return valuable feedback so that I could perfect my formulations. "Practice makes perfect," so the saying goes . . . and some of you knew when to tell me that an experimental cream, mask, or massage oil was either positively perfect or far from perfect!

Speaking of far from perfect, I remember a dreadful blueberry-mask experiment of my early years: this sweetly fragranced fruit mask, rich with beneficial antioxidants and supposedly pampering to the skin, turned a work associate's skin supremely soft — and also, regretfully, a lovely shade of pale blue. At least she had a sense of humor — thank goodness! Live, learn, and laugh, I say! Without everyone's comments and patience I could not have gained the knowledge necessary to become the natural cosmetic chemist and holistic esthetician that I am today. I thank you all.

INDEX

Page numbers in *italic* indicate photos.

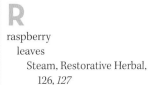

ROUND OUT YOUR
ALL-NATURAL LIBRARY
with More Books by Stephanie L. Tourles

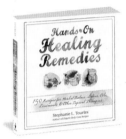

Fill your medicine cabinet with your own all-natural, topical handmade herbal remedies. More than 100 recipes for liniments, balms, and essential oil blends will help you treat a range of ailments, from arthritis to warts.

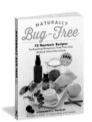

Protect yourself from mosquitoes, ticks, and other biting insects without relying on chemicals. These 75 all-natural recipes for sprays, balms, body oils, and tinctures — plus herbal pet shampoos, flea collars, and powders — are safe for your body, pets, and home.

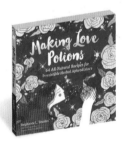

Bring some heat into your bedroom with these 64 easy recipes for herbal body oils, balms, tonics, and sweet treats. This celebration of life and pleasure includes many blends featuring familiar ingredients such as cinnamon, lavender, and vanilla.

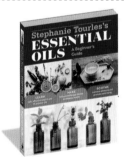

Boost your mood, relax your senses, and invigorate your mind with these 100 simple recipes. This friendly guide introduces you to the 25 most versatile essential oils, teaching you how to use these concentrated plant extracts safely and effectively.

Join the conversation. Share your experience with this book, learn more about Storey Publishing's authors, and read original essays and book excerpts at storey.com. Look for our books wherever quality books are sold or call 800-441-5700.